THE LAST 100 YEARS:
MEDICINE

THE LAST 100 YEARS:

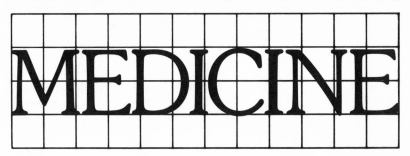

MEDICINE

DANIEL COHEN

M. Evans and Company, Inc.
New York

To Watson's Erroneous Deductions

The selections from *The Doctor's Job* by Carl Binger, M.D. that appear on pages 150-51 and 160-61 are reprinted with the permission of W. W. Norton & Company, Inc. Copyright 1945 by W. W. Norton & Company, Inc. Copyright renewed 1972 by Carl Binger.

Library of Congress Cataloging in Publication Data

Cohen, Daniel.
   The last hundred years: medicine.

   Bibliography: p.
   Includes Index.
   Summary: Highlights major developments in medicine such as the use of x-rays, certain now-common drugs, and many surgical techniques that have occurred over the last 100 years.
   1. Medicine—History—19th century—Juvenile literature. 2. Medicine—History—20th century—Juvenile literature. [1. Medicine—History] I. Title.
R149.C58   610′.9′034   81-14357

ISBN 0-87131-356-1   AACR2

M. Evans and Company, Inc.
216 East 49 Street
New York, New York 10017

Design by RONALD F. SHEY

Manufactured in the United States of America

9 8 7 6 5 4 3 2 1

CONTENTS

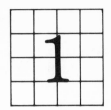

ONE HUNDRED YEARS AGO

THE CHILD HAD complained of a sore throat, and he looked flushed. When his mother put her hand to his head he felt feverish, so she sent him to bed. The mother worried, she always worried when one of her children became ill, but sore throats and fevers were common in children.

The fever grew worse, and the boy began to have difficulty breathing. The mother knew something was seriously wrong, and the doctor was sent for. He came at once, carrying his familiar black bag. The doctor was well known to the family. He had delivered the family's four children, treated their ailments and the ailments of their parents and grandparents. He was a commanding, reassuring figure.

After questioning the mother about the child's symptoms, he went to the child's bedside and said a few words to him. The boy, feverish and weak, barely responded. The doctor quickly took the boy's temperature, listened to his chest with a stethoscope, and looked down his throat with the aid of a tongue depressor. The boy choked and gagged fearfully.

By now the doctor had a pretty good idea of what condition he was dealing with, but he continued the examination, checking the boy's eyes and reflexes, pressing his stomach, feeling about his neck, and taking his pulse. The examination finished, the doctor helped the boy button up his pajama top, patted his cheek, smiled, and said that he would be fine, just fine, but that he had to stay quiet for a few days.

The doctor then snapped his black bag shut, put his arm around the mother's shoulder, and gently ushered her out of the boy's room. His smile was gone now. He looked very grave, and for good reason. His diagnosis was diphtheria. Of course, he could not be sure. The symptoms of diphtheria often looked like the symptoms of other diseases, but years of experience had given him a "feel" for such cases. Within the last week he had seen two other diphtheria cases in that very neighborhood. An epidemic seemed to be building.

The doctor told the mother to keep the boy quiet, put cold compresses on his head to relieve the fever, try to get him to take liquids—and then just wait. The gravest danger was in the next day or two, for the disease could progress rapidly, attack the heart, and death might come in a matter of hours. But even if the boy survived, it would be many months before he was truly out of danger, and even then there might be permanent damage and weakness. The doctor also advised the mother to keep her other children away from the sick boy and suggested that anything he touched be sterilized.

The doctor said that he would call in later to see how the patient was doing. He spent a few moments comforting the now weeping mother, telling her of the many similar cases he had seen in which children had recovered completely. He told the mother she must not despair, but maintain a cheerful and confident air, particularly when ministering to the sick child. The will to live, the doctor asserted, was more important than any medicine he could provide.

When the doctor finally left, he was secure in the knowledge that he had done everything he possibly could, and that he would continue to do everything he could for the difficult days and possibly months ahead. But he was also agonized by the realization that there was really very little he could do, and that he might soon be witnessing the death of a child he had brought into the world not many years before.

While the scene I have described is imaginary, it is not unlikely. Scenes like it took place frequently one hundred years ago.

One hundred years. That sounds like a long time, and in some ways it is. A lot of changes have taken place over the last hundred years, but no aspect of human life has changed more drastically than our confrontation with illness. Measured by the changes that have taken place in the world of medicine, one hundred years is not long at all. There have probably been more changes in medicine over the past hundred years than in the previous thousand years.

Let's look at the imaginary sick room again and see how it has changed. The first, and by far most important, difference is that the child-killing disease diphtheria is virtually and mercifully unknown today. It has been wiped out by medical advances.

It wasn't just diphtheria that would have frustrated our imaginary doctor of a century ago. He was nearly helpless in the face of any high fever or virulent infection. Even a simple cut might result in blood poisoning and death. The doctor's basic strategy was to let nature run its course and hope the patient survived. The modern doctor has at his command an array of medicines to fight both fevers and infection that the doctor of a century ago would have found unimaginable. There are more of these medicines than could be crammed into a dozen little black bags.

The doctor of a century ago had a thermometer, stethoscope, tongue depressor, and a few other simple instruments to help him in his diagnosis. He relied primarily on his sensitive hands and keen eyes, coupled with years of experience, to make his diagnosis. Yet even with such a well-known disease as diphtheria, diagnosis was often uncertain. In the unlikely event that a modern doctor was confronted with a suspected case of diphtheria, he would take a throat culture and send it to a laboratory for bacteriological investigation. A series of tests could confirm the diagnosis beyond any doubt.

The doctor of a century ago would have hesitated to send his patient to a hospital. For most illnesses, hospitals weren't very good, and patients received better treatment at home. Today a well-equipped hospital can provide everything from elementary nursing care for patients who do not have families that can take care of all their needs right up to total life-support systems for the gravely ill.

There have been other less obvious changes as well.

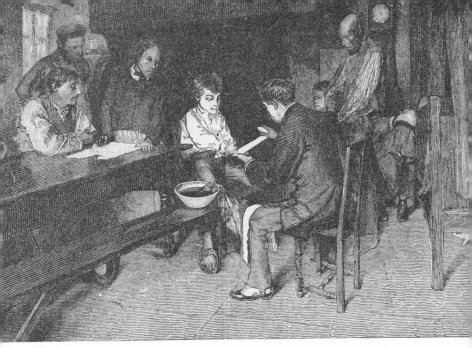

Treatment for an accident one hundred years ago and today.
(Above, New York Public Library Picture Collection)
(Below, The Johns Hopkins Medical Institutions)

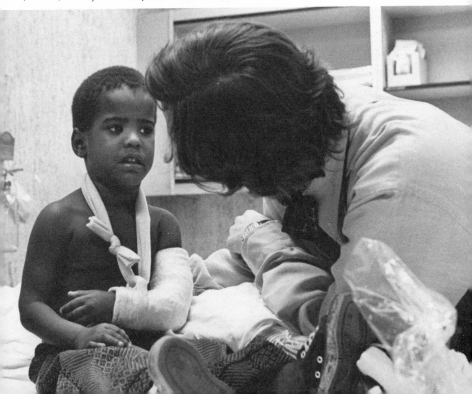

The doctor came to the sick child's home and promised to return as often as necessary. How many times have you had a doctor come to your home even once?

Our doctor of a hundred years ago had treated the entire family for a generation. There would have been no thought of sending the patient to a "specialist" even if one had been available. Today most people have their medical needs taken care of by a collection of physicians, each with a different responsibility. Most of the medical specialties of today simply did not exist one hundred years ago.

The medical world of today would be unrecognizable to the doctor and patient of one hundred years ago.

The following pages will trace the history of medicine over the last one hundred years. The changes have been so vast and complex that any attempt to provide a full history in a single small book would be a hopeless task. What we will try to do is cover some of the high points, concentrating on those changes that have had the broadest effect. A century ago there was no aspirin, and people quieted their children's coughs by filling the children full of syrups laced with opium. No one had the faintest notion what a vitamin was, and they didn't worry about high-cholesterol diets or cancer-causing chemicals in their water. Doctors still made house calls, and they were just learning to wash their hands and get out of their street clothes before performing an operation. They also might have obtained their doctor of medicine (MD) degree after less than a year of questionable training.

Traditionally, reviews of medical history are stories of relentless and inevitable progress, as medicine conquers one disease after another. In truth the story is a bit more complicated, for while progress is both undeniable and spectacular, it is more often a case of two steps forward, one back. As we shall see, there have been many wrong turns in the road of medical progress, and some of the most vexing problems that face medicine today have been created by medical progress itself.

The changes that have taken place in medicine over the last hundred years have altered not only our relationship to disease but practically everything about the way we live. It's a story with great discoveries, and mistakes, plenty of heroes, and a few villains as well.

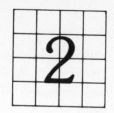

NOBEL
DISCOVERIES

WHEN ALFRED NOBEL, the immensely wealthy inventor of dynamite and other explosives, died, he left the bulk of his fortune to establish prizes for the greatest contributions in five areas of human endeavor. One of the areas was physiology and medicine. Nobel prizes have been awarded annually beginning in 1901 and have become, without a doubt, the most prestigious prizes in the world.

A list of the Nobel Prize winners and their discoveries is in many ways a summary of the most important advances in the fields of medicine and physiology for the last century. There are a couple of Nobel Prize discoveries that turned out to be dead ends, and one outright error, but by and large history has shown that the Nobel jury has chosen well.

Yet two of the most important and most publicized medical advances of the past century never received Nobel prizes in medicine. They were recognized with prizes in physics. These prizes were given to Wilhelm Röntgen for his discovery of X rays, and to Pierre and Marie Curie for their discovery of the spontaneous radiation of the element radium.

When the first Nobel prizes were awarded in 1901 no one doubted that Röntgen would get the prize for physics. Röntgen's discovery of X rays was one of the most unexpected, dramatic, and productive scientific discoveries ever. It shows that medicine does not exist in isolation from other branches of science, and particularly did not during the last century.

Röntgen, the director of the Physical Institute of the University of Würzburg in Germany, stumbled on his discovery on November 8, 1895, while experimenting with some newly developed types of vacuum tubes. Quite by accident he found that that electricity passed through a vacuum tube produced certain types of rays that were capable of penetrating dense bodies that are impenetrable by visible light rays. These rays were detected when they struck a fluorescent-coated screen and created a glow. The rays, which Röntgen called X rays because of their unknown nature, did not penetrate all dense bodies. Lead, for example was impenetrable by X rays. And when Röntgen held a piece of lead in the path of the rays he found that the rays also penetrated the flesh of his hand, yet the bones stopped some of the rays and produced an image of the skeletal hand beneath the living flesh on the fluorescent screen.

The next step was to see if the X-ray image could be captured permanently on a photographic plate. Röntgen's hunch that they could proved to be correct. The mysterious rays darkened the plate in the same way that visible light did. As the subject of the first human X-ray

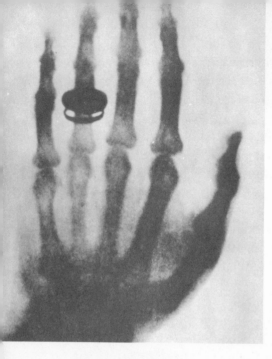

The first X-ray photograph. The hand is that of Röntgen's wife, the wedding ring clearly visible on her finger. (New York Public Library Picture Collection)

photograph Röntgen chose his wife, Birtha. She held her hand on a photographic plate while it was exposed to the rays. When the photo was developed it showed the foggy image of a skeletal hand, with a dark object covering part of the ring finger. The dark object was her wedding ring.

Röntgen seemed remarkably unimpressed by his own discovery. His only recorded comment in this period came in a letter to a friend: "I have discovered something interesting, but I do not know whether or not my observations are correct."

On December 28, 1895, Röntgen sent a paper with the deceptively simple title "On a New Kind of Rays" to the Würzburg Physical Society, and in January the discovery was announced to the world. The news of X rays was greeted with almost universal astonishment and enthusiasm. Many scientists possessed the relatively inexpensive and common equipment needed to reproduce Röntgen's experiments and to confirm that they did indeed work just as he said. Confirmation came quickly and from many sources.

The idea of rays that penetrated solid objects, including the human body, was so dramatic that the discovery captured the attention of the general public as well as the scientific community. Newspapers all over the world carried stories (often inaccurate ones) about Röntgen's X rays, and for a period the German physicist may have been the most talked about man in the world. X-ray pictures of skeletal hands and grinning skulls soon began to appear in newspaper Sunday supplements.

An X-ray photograph was something that everybody could relate to, even if they didn't really understand how it was produced. There was a popular rumor at the time that X-ray equipment could be concealed inside ordinary-looking eyeglasses. Many late-Victorian ladies feared that their modesty might be breached by this new invention. One London store announced that it was selling X-ray-proof underwear. An assemblyman named Reed from Somerset County, New Jersey, introduced a bill into the state legislature banning the manufacture or sale of X-ray opera glasses. There were also rumors of fantastic "death rays" being produced with X-ray equipment.

While physicists were fascinated by the newly discovered rays, the practical applications of the discovery to medicine became obvious almost immediately. Physicians and surgeons had suddenly and without warning been handed a diagnostic tool with which they could look inside the body. The first applications were in bone work, for the method by which Mrs. Röntgen's skeletal hand had been photographed could also be used to observe the extent of damage in a broken bone and then to see if it was set properly.

Further refinements of the process made it possible to take diagnostic X rays of internal organs, particularly of the lungs. Tuberculosis was one of the most widespread of all diseases, and in nearly 90 percent of the cases patients did not realize they had the disease until it was well advanced and infinitely more difficult to treat. Even a careful examination by a trained physician could not always detect the early signs of TB. A chest X ray could locate victims before their symptoms became acute, and wholesale screening of large segments of the population was begun.

Within a very few years after X rays were discovered no hospital was considered well equipped unless it had its own X-ray department. Physical examination usually included an X ray or fluoroscope, an instant X-ray picture that appeared on a luminous screen rather than on a photographic plate. X rays became standard in dentistry. Many shoe stores even had a type of X-ray machine with which the salesman and the customer could check the fit of a pair of new shoes.

This explosion in the use of X rays took place even though the passage of the rays through the human body is not without potential dangers, as many of the early investigators of the process discovered, often fatally. The trouble usually appeared first as chronic and painful sores on the hands and arms. These sores were resistant to all treatments and eventually turned into cancers. Some X-ray pioneers died horrible deaths after long and painful battles with cancer and many amputations. It was later discovered that X rays also increased the incidence of leukemia, as well as sterility and genetic damage. The early investigators, who had no idea of the dangers, were careless in their use of the rays and repeatedly exposed themselves to extremely high dosages. Safeguards were introduced.

As the use of X rays spread, it was realized that even the precautionary measures being taken were insufficient. Radiologists—physicians who specialize in X rays—still had an extremely high level of cancer and leukemia, and patients who were exposed to repeated doses of X rays also ran a higher risk of developing the same diseases. It wasn't until the 1960s that the full extent of the dangers from excessive X rays was appreciated.

X rays, however, were far, far too useful a tool to be abandoned. The safety of X-ray equipment was improved enormously, and procedures for operating the equipment were tightened. Unnecessary uses of X rays, for example in shoe stores, were dropped. Even mass chest X rays for tuberculosis are no longer used, because the disease is less of a danger than the X rays. In general the use of X rays is far more conservative than it was twenty or thirty years ago. Yet X rays remain one of the most significant medical advances of the last one hundred years, and it is difficult to imagine what modern medicine would be like were it not for Röntgen's accidental discovery on November 8, 1895.

The rays, which can have such a disastrous effect upon human tissue, have also been used to cure disease. Even before the turn of the century X rays were being used to treat some skin cancers, and since that time their use has been steadily extended to an increasing number of diseases, particularly various forms of cancer. At first it was hoped that the miraculous rays would provide a quick and sure cure for cancer by painlessly destroying the diseased cells. This hope turned out to be a false one, except in the case of some easily treatable skin cancers. However, X rays or X rays in conjunction with surgery and chemotherapy have been effective in retarding the growth of cancer cells, and in saving or prolonging the lives of many.

Röntgen's discovery of X rays was really the first step in the scientific exploration of radioactivity. Scientists noticed that the production of X rays in a vacuum tube was accompanied by a strong phosphorescence or glow of the glass in the tube. There are a number of substances in nature that are made phosphorescent by visible light. Therefore it seemed reasonable to suspect that these substances might emit a penetrating radiation similar to X rays. The French scientist A. H. Becquerel tested a phosphorescent compound containing the element uranium on a photographic plate wrapped in black paper. He found that the uranium fogged the plate, indicating that it emitted radiation that could penetrate materials that were opaque to ordinary light, just like X rays could.

Becquerel's discovery was followed up by the husband-and-wife team of Pierre and Marie Curie. In 1902, after a long and tedious series of experiments, they managed to isolate a new element which they named radium. It was the most radioactive substance that had ever been measured to that time. But it was rare and hard to get at. From a ton of radium-bearing ore the Curies had managed to extract a mere three-tenths of an ounce of radium itself.

Like X rays, the radiation from radium penetrated the flesh. Some of the early workers with the material found that prolonged contact produced burns on their skin. As a test, Pierre Curie bandaged a small quantity of radium to his arm. After two weeks the spot became red and blistered. After thirty days there was a deep wound that did not heal for many months. Yet the "burning" itself was painless.

An earlier medical researcher, Paul Ehrlich, had coined the term "magic bullet"—that is, a substance that would act against diseased tissue and leave healthy tissue

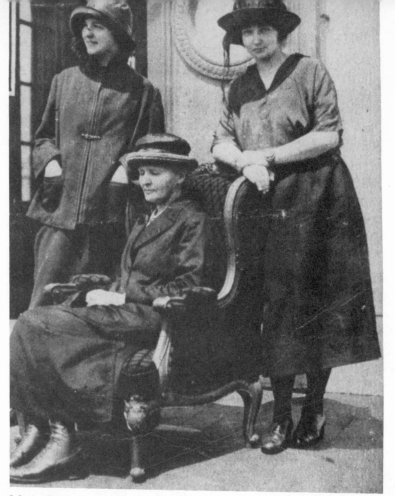

Marie Curie arrives for a tour of the United States in 1921. She is shown with her daughters Eve (left) and Irene. (Times Wide World Photos)

unharmed. As the physiological effects of radium were explored, it seemed that the substance might be just such a magic bullet for cancer. Under controlled conditions radium appeared able to destroy cancer cells without harming other tissue.

Like X rays, radium seemed miraculous, and it captured the public imagination. The Curies became world famous. Pierre Curie did not enjoy his fame for long, because in 1906 he was killed in an accident, but Marie Curie lived on to become the best-known woman scientist in history. She collected not one but two Nobel prizes for her work. Her daughter Irene also won a Nobel Prize for chemistry, and another daughter, Eve, became a well-known writer. A most remarkable family.

Radium remained difficult and expensive to produce, but the demand became so great that the price reached astronomical levels. In 1915 radium was selling at an incredible $135,000 a gram, making it the world's most expensive substance.

Radium in medicine was used in a variety of forms, as "seeds," needles, bombs, and so on. Radium was placed close to the site of a cancer in the hope that it would destroy the cancer cells. And it was useful up to a point. But radium was no magic bullet. In the end it turned out to be not nearly as effective a cancer treatment as had been hoped. With improvements in X rays and other forms of cancer therapy, the use of radium in the treatment of cancer today is virtually obsolete.

In the early years of the twentieth century, while radium was still a magic word as far as the public was concerned, a number of patent medicines were advertised as containing radium. Fortunately the advertising was false, for radium can be quite dangerous.

Like X rays, radium is capable of producing cancer as well as killing it. Workers who handled radium products in a number of different industries suffered an unusually high rate of cancer. It was years before the danger was realized and safety measures instituted or the use of radium abandoned completely.

*   *   *

Seventy years ago a diagnosis of diabetes was more feared than a diagnosis of cancer is today. Diabetes was not a new or unknown affliction. There are clear references to it in the ancient literature of Egypt, China, and India. The second-century physician Aretaeus of Cappadocia wrote of it: "Diabetes is a wonderful affection, being a melting down of the flesh into urine. . . . Life is painful and disgusting, thirst unquenchable, drinking excessive." As for treatments, there were none, and Aretaeus observed, "Death is speedy." He might have added inevitable.

By the end of the nineteenth century some understanding of diabetes had been gained. It was known to be a metabolic disorder, as a result of which the body was unable to use sugars and other food materials efficiently.

Aretaeus's description of the flesh melting into urine was dramatic though not accurate. The diabetic's rapid weight loss came about because the tissues were literally being starved, even though the patient had plenty to eat. The excessive urination was the result of the body's attempt to deal with the unmetabolized sugar, and the constant thirst was the result of dehydration due to the urination. If the disease ran its full course, in a few months or a few years the badly weakened patient would lapse into a diabetic coma and die. But the disease often did not run its course, for the diabetic is exceptionally susceptible to infection and often died of blood poisoning, pneumonia, or gangrene.

Anyone of any age might succumb to the disease, though it was most serious when it occurred in children. The expected life span of a diabetic child was less than a year. Adults might survive for ten years. The most frequent adult victims were women over forty who had a history of diabetes in their families.

In 1888 research in Germany established that diabetes was connected with the large abdominal gland, the pancreas. Previously this gland was thought to secrete only digestive juices, but it secreted something else as well, something that controlled diabetes. But what was this something else? Research into diabetes was conducted intensively for more than two decades after the German discovery, but without much success. The only treatment for the disease in 1920 was adhering to a diet so severe that the patient was left near starvation. To many victims of diabetes speedy death seemed preferable to a somewhat longer life of weakness, hunger, and the constant threat of infection.

Since researchers had begun to concentrate on the pancreas, it was virtually inevitable that someone would have eventually made the critical discovery of the substance that controlled diabetes. The man who actually did make the discovery, however, was an unlikely candidate for the honor. He was Frederick G. Banting, a shy, obscure, and not particularly well trained young Canadian physiologist. Banting had failed as a physician and had turned in desperation to teaching and research.

By 1920 researchers had come to believe that the diabetes-controlling substance was being produced by cells inside the pancreas. Banting came up with an idea that he hoped would allow him to separate the secretions of the inner cells from the strong digestive juices secreted by the outer cells of the pancreas. He didn't have the laboratory facilities, or, as he admitted, the chemical skills, to carry through an experiment to test his ideas. So he took his plan to Professor J. R. Macleod in Toronto, a distinguished medical researcher who specialized in metabolic problems. At first Macleod was wary of the totally inexperienced and rather uninformed young doctor. He turned down Banting's request for aid several times. But Banting persisted, and after a few months Macleod agreed to let Banting carry out limited experiments in his laboratory during the summer of 1921. Macleod also suggested that a young biochemist named Charles Best aid Banting with the chemical part of the work, for which Banting had no experience. Best, who usually played professional baseball in the summer, agreed to help in the lab. Macleod was going off to Scotland for a few months, and his laboratory wasn't going to be used anyway.

When Macleod returned from Scotland in the autumn, he found to his surprise that the two young men had isolated a hormone that could control the progress of diabetes in dogs. They called the substance "isletin." Macleod pointed out that that name had been used before and suggested the new discovery be called "insulin."

Once Macleod had convinced himself of the soundness of Banting's work, he put the full resources of his laboratory and his own not inconsiderable research skills behind perfecting and testing the product. There was a sense of urgency about the work. Every day people were dying of diabetes. If insulin really could control the disease, then each day of delay meant unnecessary deaths.

By January 1922, enough insulin was available in the laboratory to begin human tests. One of the first patients to receive the experimental therapy was Dr. Joe Gilchrist, a Toronto physician and an old friend of Banting. Gilchrist had developed diabetes and had reached a point in the progress of the disease where even the dietary restrictions were of little value. Without the new treatment he would not be able to survive for more than a few months. The effect that insulin injections had on Gilchrist and a few other previously doomed diabetics was nothing short of remarkable. Even the final stages of a diabetic coma could be reversed by one injection of insulin.

News of the splendid success of the treatment reached the popular press by midyear, and almost overnight Banting became a celebrity. It was a role that he did not relish or fill very well. Banting became irritable, intolerant, and just plain angry with the press. He was also deluged with requests from diabetics and their families begging to be allowed to get the new treatment, which was their only remaining hope. The vast majority of these requests had to be turned down because there simply was not enough insulin available to meet the demand. It was more than a year before there was a sufficient supply of the substance to treat more than a handful of experimental patients. Once it became available, hundreds of thousands of diabetics were suddenly given back their lives.

Normally the Nobel Prize committee moves slowly. Prizes are generally awarded for work done years earlier. The reason behind the delay is that it often takes years for the true worth of a discovery to be appreciated. But the value of insulin was so obvious and so great that the Nobel committee didn't delay at all. The very next year the prize for physiology and medicine was awarded for the discovery of insulin. It was split between two men. Banting was one, of course; the other was Macleod. Banting was furious. If anyone deserved to share the recognition, Banting insisted it was Charles Best. Macleod hadn't done anything before the discovery was made except halfheartedly lend the use of his laboratory. Banting, who was not the most tactful of men, made no attempt to hide his bitterness and announced that he was going to share his part of the prize with Best, who really should have had it anyway. Macleod was deeply offended, and a great animosity developed between the two men. Within a few years Macleod left Canada to return to Scotland forever. Banting and Best continued their researches at the University of Toronto in a medical department named after them.

On February 21, 1941, while Banting was flying to England on a war mission for the Canadian government, he was killed in a plane crash in Newfoundland.

Insulin did not provide a cure for diabetes. It merely controlled the disease, and the diabetic had to continue to take insulin for the rest of his life. Further research into diabetes has shown that it is a far more complex and widespread disease than first believed. It is now known that diabetics are prone not only to infection but to heart disease, blindness, and a host of other serious conditions.

Insulin is no longer the only treatment for diabetes. There are now a number of different drugs that are useful in mild cases. Often a carefully controlled but not starvation diet is sufficient to keep a mild case of diabetes in check.

For serious cases, and most particularly for juvenile diabetes, only insulin can do the job. Some day there may be a cure for diabetes, but today most persons who have diabetes can live nearly normal life spans with the regular use of insulin and other treatments. Even though the cause and cure of diabetes remain unknown, the outlook for victims of this once hopeless disease is hopeful indeed.

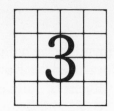

THE GREATEST VICTORIES

Epidemic diseases have brought about more major changes in world history than all the kings and generals and statesmen whose careers have been written about so often. In 1934 Hans Zinsser, a professor of bacteriology at Harvard Medical School, wrote a book with the unappealing title *Rats, Lice and History*. In this important and extremely popular study Professor Zinsser emphasized how many times the course of history had been decisively altered by an epidemic.

In Athens in 48 B.C., a plague, perhaps smallpox or typhus or a combination of diseases, so decimated and demoralized the Athenian population that it led to their ultimate defeat by Sparta and, incidentally, to the end of the Golden Age of Greece.

The Black Death, the bubonic plague, killed off anywhere from one-fourth to one-third of the population of Europe in the fourteenth century and produced profound social and political changes. Napoleon's army, badly weakened by typhus and dysentery, was routed in Russia without actually losing a battle.

More than a century ago advances in medicine and sanitation had reduced the number and severity of epidemics. Reduced them, but not eliminated them.

Yellow fever was one of those epidemic diseases that was still rampant a hundred years ago. Yellow fever or "yellow jack" was primarily a tropical disease, though there were epidemics of it regularly throughout the United States, particularly in the southern states. The worst was in 1878, when an epidemic that went up the Mississippi River as far as Memphis killed an estimated 16,000 people in a single summer.

The scenes of horror throughout the fever-ridden region rivaled those of the medieval Black Death. In cities like Memphis and New Orleans people died at the rate of one hundred a day. Caskets were carried out by the trainload. Volunteers disinfected stricken homes and burned all the blankets and bedclothing that had come in contact with the victim. Rigid quarantines were established, and those who broke the quarantine risked being shot. Yet nothing seemed to check the spread of the terrible disease until the onset of cooler weather.

A reporter for *Frank Leslie's Illustrated Newspaper*, describing the scenes of tragedy created by the epidemic, made a curious observation about the disease. He wrote of a Memphis home in which the mother had just died and the children were brought back to say good-bye: "She had the black vomit [one of the signs of the disease], and they were told they had better not kiss her, but they did, and as they came up one after the other, and gave her the last kiss on earth, their lips were stained with that horrible stream of death. And what is almost miraculous, none of them have caught the fever yet." It was another twenty years before the puzzle posed by that heartrending scene could be solved.

An earlier epidemic in Philadelphia may have had even a greater impact, for the city was less prepared. A few paragraphs from an account of the epidemic written by Mathew Carey, a Philadephia physician who observed the disease firsthand, will give you an idea of the absolute panic yellow fever could inspire:

> A woman, whose husband had just died of the fever, was seized with the pains of labour, and had nobody to assist her, as the women in the neighbourhood were afraid to go into the house. She lay for a considerable time in a degree of anguish that will not bear description. At length, she struggled to reach the window, and cried out for assistance. Two men, passing by, went upstairs; but they came at too late a stage.—She was striving with death—and actually in a few minutes expired in their arms.
>
> A woman, whose husband and two children lay dead in the room with her, was in the same situation, without a midwife, or any other person to aid her. Her cries at the window brought up one of the carters employed by the committee for the relief of the sick. With his assistance, she was delivered of a child, which died in a few minutes, as did the mother, who was utterly exhausted by her labour, by the disorder, and by the dreadful spectacle before her. And thus lay in one room no less than five dead bodies, an entire family, carried off in an hour or two.

Horrible as the disease was, the fear of it was even worse. It was fear of the unknown, for no one knew what caused the disease or how to prevent it. Most people fled the city, but those who were forced to remain were driven to desperate and extreme measures. Here is how Carey described some of them:

> Of those who remained many shut themselves up in their houses, and were afraid to walk the streets. The consumption of gunpowder and nitre in houses as a preventative was inconceivable. Many were almost incessantly purifying, scowering, and whitewashing their rooms. Those who ventured abroad had camphor, at their noses, or else smelling bottles with thieve's vinegar. Others carried pieces of tar in their hands, or pockets, or camphor bags tied round their necks. . . . People shifted their course at the sight of a hearse coming towards them. Many never walked on the foot path, but went into the middle of the streets, to avoid being infected in passing by houses wherein people had died. Acquaintances and friends avoided each other in the streets, and signified their regard by a cold nod. The old custom of shaking hands fell into such general disuse that many persons were affronted at even the offer of a hand.

Fortunately for Philadelphia and other northern cities, epidemics of yellow fever were rare. They were primarily an affliction of the South, and more particularly of the Caribbean. On an island like Cuba, yellow fever was so common that it was just part of a way of life. Most people got the disease. Some died; others survived and were immune for life. When a large number of newcomers who had never been exposed to the disease came to such an environment, they succumbed almost immediately.

Yellow fever, malaria, and other tropical diseases had very nearly defeated the American troops in the Spanish-American War. The small and ill-equipped Spanish forces were no match for the Americans. Had the Spanish been able to hold on just a bit longer, however, the disease-wracked American army would have been forced to withdraw. As it was, the U.S. casualties from the fighting were almost negligible, while the disease toll was appalling.

In 1899 the United States found itself in temporary possession of the fever-ridden island of Cuba. This raised the specter of disease ravaging the American military occupation forces. But if yellow fever could be reduced or eliminated in Cuba, this presented the opportunity of attacking one of the main strongholds of the disease and thus, it was hoped, reducing the constant menace to the South.

The cause of yellow fever was unknown in 1899. It was simply assumed that improved sanitary conditions would either eradicate or sharply reduce the incidence of yellow fever, as such improvements had already done for so many other deadly diseases. Havana was then a filthy city. It had only one or two sewers, and garbage was just thrown into the narrow streets. Sanitary conditions in Havana had never been very good, and at this time they were worse than ever because of the disruptions caused by the long Cuban insurrection and the American invasion.

The task of cleaning up the city was given to an army surgeon, Major William Crawford Gorgas. With strong backing from his superior, Major General Leonard Wood, who was the governor general of Cuba, Gorgas did an astonishingly good job in just a few months. From a rubbish-filled city in decay, Havana became cleaner than most American cities of the period. At first Gorgas's cleanup seemed to do the job on yellow fever. Reported cases fell sharply through 1899. But by 1900 the number of cases was on the rise, and shortly there was a full-scale epidemic raging once again. The improvements in sanitation had not the slightest effect on yellow fever.

What had happened was that yellow fever had been so prevalent in Havana that practically everyone had had the disease, and the survivors were immune. In December 1899 some 12,000 Spanish peasants arrived in Cuba. They were not immune and became the main sufferers in the new epidemic. Yellow fever had not been destroyed or even dented. It had simply lacked suitable victims. When they arrived, it came back in full force.

Yellow fever is a horrible disease. It begins suddenly with painful headaches and backaches and a rapidly rising fever. Nausea and persistent vomiting follow. If the case is a severe one there is a great deal of internal bleeding, and the vomiting of dark altered blood gives the disease its Spanish name, *el vómito negro*—black vomit. The English name, yellow fever, comes from a yellowing of the skin and eyes that takes place in many victims. This is a side effect, for the disease destroys liver cells and causes jaundice, which in turn produces the yellowing.

The more seriously afflicted die within a few days. Even relatively mild cases kill the very young, the elderly, or those who are already in a weakened condition. For the survivors there is a long period of convalescence, and sometimes permanent damage, as well as a lifelong immunity.

The disease could create enormous problems for nonimmune North Americans sent to Cuba. Small wonder, then, that after the high hopes of 1899 the return of yellow fever in 1900 produced a great deal of angry shouting and finger pointing in Washington. Everybody demanded that something be done. The government responded by appointing a commission of four army surgeons, headed by Dr. Walter Reed.

The task of tracking down and eradicating yellow fever was made particularly difficult and dangerous because no known laboratory animal could contract it. If experiments were needed, they would have to be done in the field on human beings. In many respects yellow fever was, or appeared to be, a peculiar disease. It did not seem to be contagious, that is, spread directly from person to person as, for example, smallpox. Yet it undoubtedly did spread, through the action of some unknown agency.

There were two directions that Dr. Reed and his associates might explore. The first was to try to identify the yellow fever "germ" itself and then develop either an innoculation that would prevent the disease or an antitoxin that would cure it. In 1897 an Italian researcher announced that he had isolated the bacillus that caused yellow fever. The announcement was greeted with enthusiasm in medical circles in the United States. Before being appointed to the yellow fever commission, Reed had already been hard at work trying to confirm the Italian research, but he was unable to do so. He became convinced that the 1897 Italian announcement was an error.

A second direction for research was to forget about the cause of the disease and concentrate on the means by which it was spread. It was this second approach that Reed and his associates decided to pursue. A fortunate decision, for yellow fever is caused not by a bacillus but by a far smaller virus, which proved to be extraordinarily difficult to locate. It was nearly thirty years after the appointment of the Reed commission that the specific viral cause of yellow fever was identified and an effective innoculation developed. By that time the disease was no longer a major threat because the means by which it spread had been found and effectively dealt with.

In 1900 one popular theory was that yellow fever was spread by fomites—a Latin word rather vaguely meaning substances capable of transmitting contagion. These fomites might be found in the clothing, bedding, or anything else that had been in close contact with the yellow fever victim.

To test the fomite theory, the Reed commission had three volunteers spend twenty-one days sleeping on sheets and under blankets that had been taken directly from the yellow fever hospital in Havana. The sheets were literally stiff with the black vomit of the sick. The men spent their nights locked in a tiny, almost airless cabin with their reeking bedclothes. The days were spent in the boredom of an isolation tent. The aim of this tight supervision was not only to keep in the fomites, if such things existed, but to screen out other possible sources of yellow fever infection. After twenty-one hot, stinking, and airless nights and twenty-one worrisome days, the men were released from quarantine. Not one of them had developed yellow fever. Later volunteers slept in the very pajamas used by disease victims or in sheets soaked in their blood. If fomites existed, there should have been enough of them in this sort of material to infect a city, yet not one of these volunteers came down with yellow fever.

For some twenty years a Cuban physician, Dr. Carlos Finlay, had been quietly insisting that the agent for transmission of yellow fever was a particular type of mosquito,

Aedes aegypti. He had never been able to prove his theory. As a result he had come to be regarded as something of a medical eccentric with a strange obsession. Perhaps out of desperation as much as anything else, Reed decided to test Finlay's mosquito hypothesis. Reed himself was immune to yellow fever, having had a mild case earlier in his career. But Drs. James Carroll and Jesse Lazear were not immune, and they served as guinea pigs in the experiment. Both contracted yellow fever after being bitten by mosquitoes that had fed on the blood of yellow fever victims. Lazear died within a few days, and Carroll was so severely weakened by the disease that his life was greatly shortened. Both men were hailed as martyrs to humanity, which indeed they were.

Still, the mosquito bites and the onset of the disease might have been coincidental. Experiments under more controlled conditions were needed to prove the mosquito connection. In an open, uncultivated field near Havana, an experimental sanitary station, named after Dr. Lazear, was established on November 20, 1900. Half the subjects of the experiment were poor Spanish immigrants who were attracted by a payment of $250. The rest were young volunteers from the U.S. military forces. The first to subject himself to the bite of an infected mosquito and to get the disease was Private John R. Kissinger. Though he became gravely ill, he recovered. Other subjects, both American and Spanish, came down with the disease with such predictable regularity that it was possible to determine the exact conditions under which yellow fever was transmitted by the mosquito.

While the doctors and volunteers who had participated in this epochal discovery were hailed as heroes and martyrs, the U.S. government treated them very shabbily.

Carroll's and Lazear's widows were forced to scrape along on small pensions. Reed died in 1902 of appendicitis. (Ironically, this medical pioneer could have been saved by a prompt and simple operation.) His widow did not receive anything from the government until twenty-one years after his death. Poor Kissinger had an even worse time. His health was broken, and after he left the army he became a paralytic. His wife both nursed and supported him until 1907, when in recognition of his services to humanity he was granted a pension of $12 a month! Finally, in 1922, an embarrassed Congress raised his pension to $100 a month.

Once the transmission by mosquito was recognized, the nearly complete eradication of yellow fever in Havana was quickly and easily accomplished. This was because of a peculiarity of the habits of the carrier *Aedes aegypti* mosquito. There are hundreds of varieties of mosquitoes. Most of them live in swamps, lay their eggs in stagnant water, and can range over a wide area. Such an insect is difficult to control. *Aedes aegypti* was peculiarly domesticated. It preferred to live in houses and lay its eggs in clean water, found in water barrels, cisterns, pitchers, or some other domestic utensil. Cuba was still under U.S. military occupation, and Major Gorgas, who had cleaned up Havana with such efficiency, now set out to "get rid of the mosquito."

His inspectors roamed the streets and thoroughly searched every house for places in which the mosquito could breed. Larger deposits of water were covered with a film of oil to smother the mosquito larva. Housewives were compelled to produce every single receptacle capable of holding water. Penalties for noncompliance were severe. It was the sort of campaign that could have been carried out only under military rule. And it worked. Cases of yellow fever began to fall rapidly, until finally, for the first time in centuries, there were none in Havana.

The eradication of yellow fever was to have almost immediate political effects. Many nations had dreamed of building a canal across the isthmus of Panama to connect the Atlantic and Pacific oceans and cut down the long voyage around the tip of South America. In the early 1880s Ferdinand de Lesseps, who built the Suez Canal, formed a French corporation to dig a canal across Panama. When digging actually began, the work force was so weakened by the effects of yellow fever, malaria, and other tropical diseases that the attempt ended in a costly and tragic failure.

By the turn of the century, America, emboldened by its success in the Spanish-American War, determined to build its own Panama Canal. Gorgas was put in charge of sanitation, but he was not given the necessary power to launch an effective anti-mosquito campaign. By 1905 there was a yellow fever epidemic raging in the towns along the proposed canal. Many in government and the military still did not believe in the mosquito transmission of disease theory, and they urged that Gorgas be dismissed. Finally President Theodore Roosevelt came out on Gorgas's side, and Gorgas was given a free hand to eradicate the mosquito in Panama.

In September 1905, a buoyant Gorgas entered the dissecting room of the government hospital at Ancon, where a number of surgeons were dissecting the corpse of a yellow fever victim.

"Take a good look at this man, boys," he told the surgeons, "for it's the last case of yellow fever you will ever see. There will never be any more deaths from this cause in Panama."

A confident assertion, and a correct one as it turned out. The scourge of tropical regions has been reduced to a medical curiosity. In regions where it was once common, many doctors today have never even seen a case of the disease.

The almost complete conquest of yellow fever is one of the happiest medical success stories of the last century, but it is certainly not the only one. Medicine has had enormous success against other infectious diseases, particularly those that afflicted children. Complete protection against the deadly and disfiguring disease smallpox had been developed during the early years of the nineteenth century through the work of Dr. Edward Jenner. Today smallpox has been virtually eliminated from the world, and the smallpox vaccinations that not long ago were a part of every child's life are no longer considered necessary. Smallpox is the first disease to be declared extinct. The germ theory, which held that many diseases were caused by microorganisms, and the scientific principle behind innoculation were developed more than a century ago.

Even with smallpox out of the way, the late-nineteenth-century child faced the dangers of diphtheria, whooping cough, and scarlet fever, any one of which could result in a painful death. The first effective protection against diphtheria, an antitoxin, was developed in the 1890s. Treatments were steadily improved over the next thirty years, until virtually complete immunity to the disease could be obtained by a series of injections. A vaccine for whooping cough, or pertussis, was first introduced in

1914. And yet every year thousands of children throughout the world continue to die of these preventable diseases, either because the proper vaccines were not available or because people simply failed to take advantage of them. In many of the industrialized nations of the world immunization was made compulsory, and the results were often dramatic. In the decade from 1910 to 1919 there were 14,282 cases of diphtheria in New York City, with 1,290 deaths as an annual average. Then diphtheria immunization was made compulsory before the admission of children to school. In 1942 there were 413 cases, with 7 deaths. Today both diphtheria and whooping cough are medical rarities in the industrialized nations, and intensive campaigns by the World Health Organization and other international bodies are reducing the incidence of these diseases in the less-developed parts of the world.

The first innoculation that most children receive, at the age of about two months, is called DPT. It contains vaccines for diphtheria, pertussis, and tetanus. Tetanus, or lockjaw, is a serious disease, but not contagious. It is contracted directly when tetanus bacteria enter the skin through a wound. Two or three boosters for diphtheria and pertussis are given to children under the age of five, and this is usually enough to confer lifetime immunity. Tetanus boosters are given more frequently, and they are also administered when a person steps on a rusty nail, is bitten by a dog, or has some other possible exposure to the bacteria.

Scarlet fever is another matter. For reasons that are not really understood, the severity of the disease has declined sharply in recent times. Fifty years ago scarlet fever victims were quarantined, and parents feared that the disease would lead to heart-damaging rheumatic fever. Today

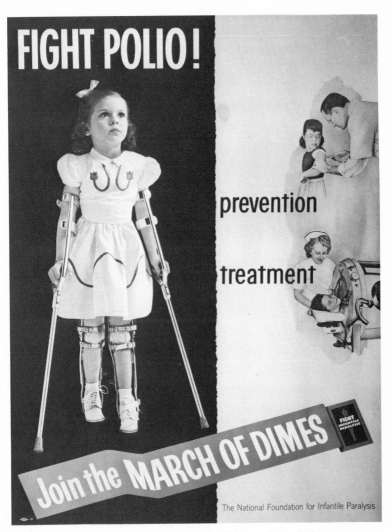

A March of Dimes poster. (*The March of Dimes Foundation*)

ACUTE ANTERIOR POLIOMYELITIS

(*A COMMUNICABLE DISEASE*)

Keep Out of this House   By Order of BOARD OF HEALTH

HEALTH OFFICER

Any person removing this card without authority is liable to prosecution.

Polio quarantine poster used in 1910. (The National Library of Medicine)

scarlet fever is a relatively mild infection, easily and effectively treated with antibiotics. No one knows why scarlet fever is less virulent now than half a century ago. It is a reminder that despite the great advances against infectious diseases there is a great deal that we still don't know about them.

As each of these childhood dangers was eliminated or reduced, medical science took aim at a new target. During the 1950s the target was polio, a disease that could result in death but more often crippled its victims. President Franklin D. Roosevelt was stricken as an adult and completely lost the use of his legs. Throughout his terms as president, and he held the office longer than anyone else in history, he was pushed about in a wheelchair and could stand only with the aid of metal leg braces. Oddly, although everyone knew he was crippled, no issue was ever made of it. Photographers never showed President Rooseveld in his wheelchair or being carried into his limousine. It was a subject that everyone knew about but no one talked about.

There was certainly plenty of talk about polio itself. The March of Dimes, one of the most successful fundraising efforts in the history of American charities, has the eradication of polio as its main goal. Everyone was aware of the annual "poster child," a brave, severely crippled victim of the disease, smiling appealingly while supporting himself or herself with crutches and braces. And there was a terrifying image—the iron lung. This was a coffinlike machine in which totally paralyzed polio victims had to spend their lives, just so that they could keep breathing.

There were some who said that all the publicity had generated an exaggerated dread of polio. Yes, there was no doubt it was a serious disease that could kill and cripple, but there were many serious diseases that were being approached more calmly. For many children an attack of polio was so mild that it left no aftereffects, and might even go undetected. Most children probably had polio without knowing it. Besides, said the critics, the virulence of polio appeared to be on the decline, and without any medical intervention at all the disease was becoming less serious. Appeals to calm were not heard in the polio-conscious 1950s. The merest hint of a "polio epidemic" would cause parents to keep their children off the beaches, out of the movie theatres and other public places for an entire summer.

The virus that caused the disease had been identified, and it was only a matter of developing an adequate and safe vaccine. Enormous professional, personal, and financial rewards awaited the developer of the first safe polio vaccine. The work of different researchers took on the almost frantic quality of a race. The winner of the race was Dr. Jonas Salk of New York. His polio vaccine was given mass public tests in 1954 and approved for general use in 1955. Salk's vaccine produced immunity through the use of polio viruses that had been killed. Two years later Dr.

Albert Sabin came out with a vaccine that used viruses that were still alive but had been weakened to the point where they produced the immunity without the disease. Sabin claimed that his vaccine was more effective and easier to administer. While the Salk vaccine had to be injected, the Sabin vaccine could be taken orally, usually by putting a couple of drops on a cube of sugar. The Salk vaccine continued to be most popular in America, while the Sabin vaccine was used widely in Europe and ultimately became the favored form of innoculation in the United States as well. There was, and still is, a controversy between the supporters of these two different approaches to vaccines. But this meant nothing to the general public. Within a few years after the introduction of the first polio vaccine, and after intensive publicity campaigns aimed at getting every child vaccinated, polio had been reduced from a dread disease to a rare one. Children born after 1955 no longer had to face the summer polio panics.

After the near eradication of the polio menace, attention was focused on the remaining childhood infectious diseases. Mumps produced a painful swelling of glands in the neck and jaw. Cartoonists commonly showed the mumps sufferer with horribly swollen cheeks and a bandage wrapped loosely around his head. The disease was no laughing matter to the child who had it, but after the discomfort there were rarely any lasting complications. For adults it was a different matter. If a person managed to avoid the disease, and thus immunity to it, until he was older, an attack of mumps might produce serious aftereffects, even death. One of the most common results of adult mumps was sterility in men. For this reason many parents took no special precautions to keep their children from getting mumps, and some deliberately exposed chil-

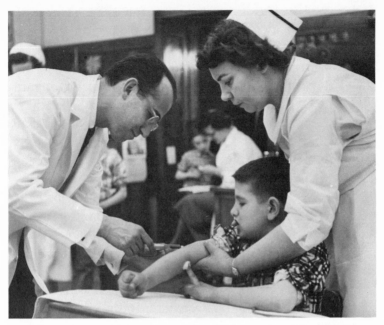

Dr. Jonas Salk giving an injection of his polio vaccine. (The March of Dimes Foundation)

dren to the disease. Better discomfort while young than the risk of serious damage when older. Better still was a vaccine that produced no symptoms, but would produce immunity. Such a vaccine was developed in 1964.

Measles is a disease that produces high fevers and unsightly skin eruptions and occasionally weakens a young patient so severely that he or she is prone to more serious secondary infections. The development of antibiotics cut the risk of serious secondary infections, but measles was still a disease to be avoided. A measles vaccine was developed by 1963. Yet measles is still with us. It is not that the measles vaccine is not effective—it is very effective. The problem is that many children have not been immunized.

It may be that because the disease is not considered to be too serious, many parents are lax in making sure that their children have been innoculated. The result is persistent localized measles epidemics. One child in a community gets the disease, and suddenly a large number of his nonimmune schoolmates and friends come down with it. This usually prompts local health officials to initiate a strict compulsory innoculation campaign—no measles shots, no school.

By 1981 the campaign against measles had been so successful that officials of the Federal Centers for Disease Control predicted that the disease would soon be eliminated in the United States. Rubella and mumps had also decreased significantly in 1981.

German measles, or rubella, is an extremely mild childhood disease that carries with it a hidden danger. In a child or most nonimmune adults, rubella is hardly worse than a bad cold. But if a woman gets the disease in the early months of pregnancy, the results can be catastrophic. The virus attacks the unborn child and can produce severe birth defects. Epidemics of German measles were inevitably followed by a sharp rise in the number of birth defects. A rubella vaccine was developed in the late 1960s, and since that time the damage done by this cruelly insidious disease has been sharply reduced.

Whooping cough, diphtheria, scarlet fever, polio, measles, mumps, and rubella, all of the major childhood infectious diseases of the past one hundred years, have either been eliminated or severely reduced as menaces. The only old-style childhood disease that remains is chicken pox, and while it is both ugly and uncomfortable, it is not a dangerous disease. It is probably the only one of these childhood diseases (with the exception, perhaps, of a mild case of scarlet fever) that you have ever had.

Other infectious diseases like cholera, typhoid, and malaria, which were once responsible for major epidemics, have now been successfully controlled, primarily by public health measures like water purification. Bubonic plague, the feared Black Death of the Middle Ages, is now so rare that a recent suspected case in New York City sent the doctors scurrying to their old medical reference works. In the end, the patient was cured so quickly and completely that the doctors never could be sure that's what he had in the first place. That is all that remains today of the feared plague.

Another of the human race's ancient enemies, tuberculosis, often called TB, consumption, or the white plague, has not been so successfully combated. It is reasonable to suggest that tuberculosis has killed and disabled more people over a longer period than any other disease in history. Until 1909 it was the leading cause of death in the United States. Usually the disease kills slowly and painfully by destroying the lungs. So many well-known artists, writers, and musicians died of tuberculosis that for a time there was almost a romantic aura attached to it. It was theorized that somehow the fever that accompanied the disease was a stimulus to creativity. Some people even affected having tuberculosis and carried about a handkerchief into which they coughed frequently. The facts are far grimmer. The real victims would eagerly have traded the supposed creative spur of tuberculosis to be free of the disease.

The actual cause of TB, the *tubercle bacillus*, was discovered by the great bacteriologist Robert Koch of Germany in 1882. But unlike for some bacteria-caused diseases, it was not easy to develop an effective antituberculosis vaccine. Nor has the disease proved easy to control through relatively straightforward sanitary measures, as in the case of yellow fever. The most common TB victims are those who live under crowded conditions and may already be weakened because of poor nutrition and other diseases. In short, the people who most commonly suffer from tuberculosis are the poor. While excellent treatments for tuberculosis are now available, poverty is still with us, and TB still afflicts far more people than it should, even in the United States. The persistence of tuberculosis remains a medical and social scandal.

Influenza, or the flu, is the most widespread infectious disease in the world today. Most of us regard a case of the flu, with its fever, chills, body aches, and coughing, as an uncomfortable, inconvenient interlude, but nothing more. Yet flu can be serious, particularly to the elderly or to those who already suffer from some sort of respiratory ailment. Much also depends on the virulence of the particular kind of flu, for there are many different types of flu virus.

The most deadly epidemic of modern times was the outbreak of what was called Spanish Influenza at the end of World War I in 1918. It caused half a million deaths in the United States alone, and perhaps twenty million worldwide. In terms of lives lost, it was more deadly than the Great War itself. Every few years there is another worldwide flu epidemic, and some, like the Hong Kong flu of 1968–69, have been quite severe, though none have come near matching the deadly toll of the Spanish Influenza.

The human influenza virus was first isolated in 1933 and has been the subject of intensive study ever since. Why, then, do we have no effective protection against it? Why do we still face getting the flu every few years? There are

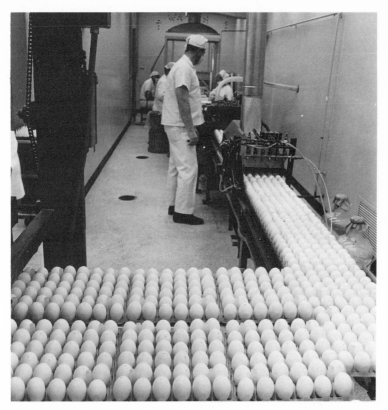

Vaccine for the influenza virus is incubated in fresh fertile eggs. (Warner-Lambert Company)

several reasons. Since flu symptoms resemble the symptoms of a number of other respiratory diseases, we often think we have the flu when in fact we have something else. More significantly, however, influenza is caused not by a single virus but by many types of closely related viruses. Moreover, from time to time entirely new types of flu virus appear. After suffering through one type of flu, a person may become immune to it but still be vulnerable to infection by another type.

Typically, a worldwide flu epidemic, or pandemic, begins in one place, and because it is highly contagious, travelers soon carry it to other parts of the world, where new local outbreaks begin. The pattern ends only when most of the world's population has become immune to that particular type of flu virus.

There are vaccines for the various strains of flu, but there are so many different types of influenza virus that you can never be sure you are being vaccinated for the right one. During a major epidemic the vaccine cannot be produced quickly enough, so by the time the vaccine is available most susceptible individuals have already had the disease. Even if you get the right vaccine in time, you may still get the flu, because the vaccines are not 100 percent effective.

Then you must remember that every medical treatment, including immunization, carries with it some risk of complications or side effects. A striking example of the complexities and problems associated with flu innoculation can be seen in what happened during the winter of 1975–76. A flu epidemic broke out in China and began to spread rapidly. This particular type of flu was called swine flu because it was thought that the virus had originally infected pigs. Experts in communicable diseases determined that the swine flu virus was virtually identical to the virus that had produced the horrible Spanish flu pandemic of 1918. Most people alive at the time had been born since 1918, so the vast majority of the world's population had no immunity to the swine flu virus.

Some medical authorities in the United States had grim visions of a repeat of the 1918 killer epidemic, and they urged a crash program to produce great quantities of vaccine to innoculate as many people as possible before the disease struck in full force. The vaccine was produced, but the innoculation program turned out to be a total failure and something of a joke, although at times a rather unfunny one.

The predicted severe epidemic never materialized. Swine flu was both milder and less contagious than anticipated. Lots of people were innoculated, and as in every mass innoculation program, there were a small number of adverse reactions, including several cases of a rare but severe type of paralysis, associated with the innoculation. Had there really been a serious influenza epidemic raging, these bad reactions would hardly have been noticed. With no epidemic to speak of, press and public attention concentrated on the adverse reactions, and the entire swine flu innoculation program was discredited. Whether it should have been started at all is still a matter of controversy.

So each time a new type of flu makes its appearance, people wonder, "Should I get flu shots?" Most of the time they don't.

Looking back over a century of attack on epidemic diseases, from the stunning success in the control of yellow fever to the ambiguous success of the flu shots, medical science can be well satisfied. Perhaps some of the claims of success have been a bit exaggerated, but exaggeration is entirely pardonable in this area. Most bacteria or virus-caused diseases feared by our parents and grandparents have been either eliminated or sharply reduced, particularly in the area of childhood diseases. Were it not for these successes, a large percentage of us would not have lived long enough to be able to worry about heart disease, cancer, and the other diseases of maturity and old age.

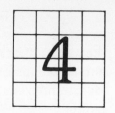

THE KING'S
APPENDIX

In June 1902 all London was decorated for the coronation of King Edward VII. The coronation was a long-anticipated event. For many years it had seemed as if the new king's formidable mother, Queen Victoria, would live forever, but in January 1901 she finally died. Her son, now sixty, overweight from too much eating and wheezy from too much smoking, ascended the throne. His coronation, however, was not scheduled until June of the following year.

The event was not merely an English ceremony, it was eagerly awaited throughout the world. In 1902 England was the most powerful nation on earth. Its empire and commonwealth stretched to all parts of the globe. London was jammed with visitors hoping to catch a glimpse of the pomp and grandeur that accompanied the great event.

Then on June 24, just a day before the scheduled coronation, while rehearsals were actually being held in

Westminster Abbey, came a shocking announcement. The coronation of Edward VII was to be posponed indefinitely because the king was ill and needed an operation. According to the official bulletin: "The King is undergoing a surgical operation. The King is suffering from perityphlitis. His condition on Saturday was so satisfactory that it was hoped that with care His Majesty would be able to go through the Coronation Ceremony. On Monday evening a recurrence became manifest, rendering a surgical operation necessary today."

In other words, the king was having his appendix removed. The king's condition was serious, and even after the operation was successfully performed, there were many anxious and uncertain days. The doctors waited to see if the king would develop general peritonitis, a usually fatal infection that often followed such operations. There were any number of other serious complications that could have set in, particularly considering the king's age and condition. But luck was with Edward VII. His fever began to go down and he recovered rapidly and completely. Twenty years earlier he would have died in lingering agony, as did Léon Gambetta, the premier of France. Gambetta had the same condition as Edward. He expired on December 31, 1882, after a month of suffering that was in no way relieved by the constant attentions of Europe's leading physicians.

Had the king been a simple American workingman in 1902, however, his condition probably would never have been allowed to deteriorate so badly. His appendix would have been removed by a simple procedure, that had already become commonplace in America. English physicians, however, distrusted the radical surgical technique developed in America. To be fair to them, their patient also distrusted the treatment, and he was, after all, king of England. Edward was not used to obeying doctors' orders, or anybody's orders but his own.

The king's acute symptoms began to appear on the thirteenth, eleven days before the operation. He complained of pain and intense nausea. The king was forced to curtail some of his activities, and the standard treatments, including large doses of opium, didn't seem to be helping much. It wasn't until the eighteenth that the king's doctor decided surgery might be necessary, but when this was mentioned to the king he went into a rage and ordered his physician out of the room. Edward VII was not afraid of the operation, but he didn't want all the preparations for the coronation ruined. Edward VII was a man to whom ceremony was very important.

The symptoms persisted and grew worse. Finally, on the twenty-fourth, the king's physician, Sir Francis Laking, simply refused to leave the room when he was ordered out. He continued to insist that an immediate operation was essential or else, quite simply, the king would die. Edward finally gave way. An operating room in the palace had already been prepared. The chief surgeon, Frederick Treves, found that the appendix had already burst and that there was a major area of infection, but so far at least the infection had not spread. The abscess was drained, and in forty minutes it was all over, except for waiting to see if the infection had been caught in time.

For hundreds of years physicians had helplessly watched their patients die of mysterious "abdominal affections on the right side." Vomiting and fever were followed by signs of severe intestinal inflammation, general peritoni-

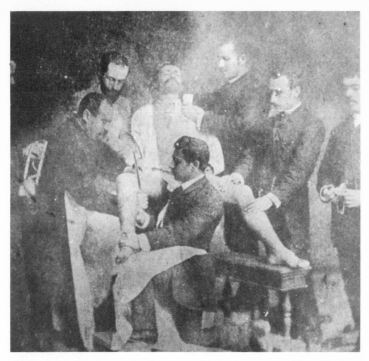

Surgery in the preanesthetic era could be gruesome. (New York Public Library Picture Collection)

tis, and usually death. Occasionally a patient recovered, but the ordeal was a frightful one. None of the usual treatments for abdominal "affections" seemed to work, and they often appeared to make the patient worse. What all of these unfortunates suffered from was an inflammation of the appendix, a tiny attachment to the part of the intestine known as the blind gut.

Before the middle of the nineteenth century, any attempt to remove an inflamed appendix surgically, even if it was thought necessary, would have been tantamount to murder. Two developments changed that. The first was the use of anesthetics—substances that rendered the patient unconscious or otherwise insensible to pain. Before anesthesia any surgery—and it was mainly amputations or the repair of traumatic wounds—was a horror show. Patients screamed themselves into insensibility and often died of shock from the pain of the operation. Strength and speed, not delicacy or skill, were the surgeon's greatest assets. The nearly legendary hero of the preanesthetic era was the British surgeon Sir Robert Liston, who could amputate a patient's leg at the thigh in thirty-three seconds, according to the *Guiness Book of World Records*. Said one of his admiring colleagues, "The gleam of his knife was followed so swiftly by the sound of sawing as to make the two actions appear almost simultaneous." Liston worked at such a frenzied speed that during one operation he accidentally amputated three of his assistant's fingers.

Anesthetics changed all of that. But surgery remained a desperate gamble, for the patient was very likely to die from postsurgical infection. That too changed with the introduction of antisepsis—simply keeping the wound and the surgical instruments clean and as germ free as possible.

Both of these monumental improvements were accepted by about 1850, yet an operation for an inflamed appendix would still have been impossible, because no one knew that the tiny appendix was where the infection started. Even with anesthetics and antiseptic surgery, opening the abdomen was still a traumatic event, and one to be carried out as rarely as possible. When a surgeon did finally operate on a patient with an inflammation on the lower right side, it was only after the infection had become extremely serious. By then the appendix had usually burst and the infection had become general. Either the tiny appendix was overlooked or everyone assumed that the inflammation of the appendix had been the result of a disease that had started in the bland gut—the reverse of the real situation. The name "perityphlitis" was given to this condition. It meant roughly "inflammation in this area of the intestine." The name itself created a problem because it ignored the appendix completely. The appendix was so small, so useless, that doctors just didn't look for problems to start there.

All this began to change in 1886, when an anatomist and pathologist in Boston announced that he had dissected more than five hundred persons who had died in various stages of perityphlitis. In almost all of these cases he found that the inflammation had begun in the appendix. He suggested that the name of the disease be changed from perityphlitis to "appendicitis," "inflammation of the appendix," which more truly described the condition.

The anatomist was Reginald Heber Fitz, a German who had emigrated to America and become professor of pathological anatomy at Harvard Medical School. Fitz was known to be a fanatic about dissection. According to one tale, Fitz went to visit a friend who was ill. But he stared at the sick man with such a glassy-eyed look that the poor fellow was terror stricken. He thought the fanatic dissector was going to begin an autopsy on him, even though he wasn't dead.

Fanatic or not, Fitz had not only correctly located the origin of the problem but suggested the right treatment. The surgeon must not limit himself to opening the abscesses once the infection became impossible to ignore. He must remove the inflamed appendix at the earliest possible moment. Surgeons at first reacted a bit like Fitz's sick

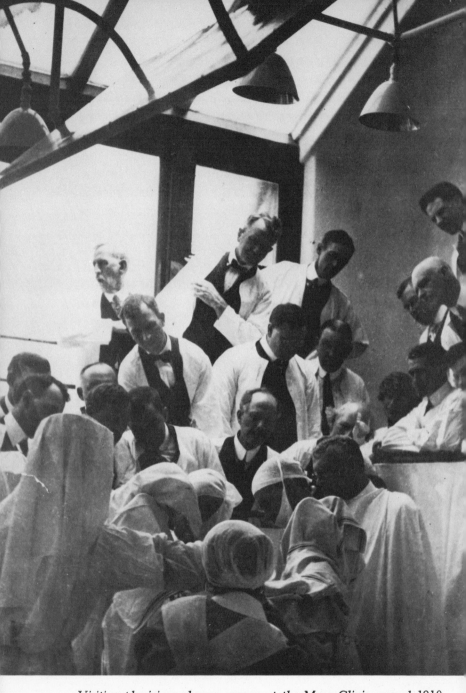

*Visiting physicians observe surgery at the Mayo Clinic around 1910.
(The Mayo Clinic)*

friend. They thought the anatomist was mad; to open a patient's abdomen before his life was actually in danger seemed the height of folly. But after a few years some surgeons tried the operation on their patients and it worked —suffering was cut short and many lives were saved.

By the turn of the century, operations to remove an inflamed appendix were fairly commonplace in America, and reasonably safe as well. In Europe, however, the old view of perityphlitis hung on, and the surgeon was called in only after the infection had become so serious that the abscess had to be drained. By then the patient's life was in grave and immediate peril. That was the situation that had faced King Edward VII. His doctors had not quite accepted the new appendicitis operation, and as a result they very nearly killed their king.

The operation to remove an inflamed appendix before it became a serious problem caught on and ultimately became something of a medical fad. The removal of the appendix became almost routine. In the opinion of some medical authorities, appendectomies were often done without sufficient reason. While the average, appendectomy is a low-risk operation, no surgical procedure is entirely without danger. It is generally considered wise and prudent to avoid surgery whenever possible. Critics of the extensive use of the appendectomy pointed out that even before the introduction of the operation most of those who suffered from a mildly inflamed appendix recovered anyway. What with antibiotics and other drugs, less drastic remedies than surgery were available. Surgery, said the critics, should be reserved for more serious cases. The critics made telling points, and today the operation to remove an inflamed appendix, while still common, is far less common than it was twenty or thirty years ago.

Since even the simplest operation carries some risk and is usually irreversible, surgery has always been one of the more controversial areas of medicine. Despite the almost miraculous advances in surgery during the past century there has been a constant undercurrent of complaint that some surgery, perhaps a great deal of it, is excessive and unnecessary.

The playwright George Bernard Shaw was no friend of the medical profession. But he made some telling points in his play *The Doctor's Dilemma*, particularly in his parody of the popularity of the appendectomy. One of the characters, a surgeon named Cutler Walpole, believes that 95 percent of the human race is suffering from blood poisoning because of an infected "nuciform sac."

"I tell you this," says the surgeon. "In an intelligently governed country people wouldn't be allowed to go about with nuciform sacs, making themselves centres of infection. The operation ought to be compulsory: It's ten times more important that vaccination."

Excessive and unnecessary were the objections raised against what was once far and away the most common operation in America, the tonsillectomy, removal of tonsils. The tonsils are masses of lymph tissue in the throat. Their purpose is to act as a barrier against bacterial infection, but they often become the centers of infection. Fevers, sore throats, or other symptoms due to inflamed or enlarged tonsils were reported frequently. Starting in the 1880s there was one sure cure proposed for inflamed tonsils, or tonsillitis—take out the tonsils. For good measure the nearby adenoids were usually removed as well. The operation was not merely common, it was routine, practically mandatory. Doctors regarded tonsils the way Cutler Walpole regarded the "nuciform sac." Children from the ages of about four to twelve who suffered from sore throats or were thought to be "mouth breathers" were taken off to the hospital for a tonsillectomy. It was the first and sometimes the only operation a child would ever have. The experience of entering a hospital could be a frightening one, but the young patients were always promised that afterward they could eat all the ice cream they wanted. What they were not told was that for several days their throats would be so sore they could eat nothing else.

The vogue for removing tonsils, which began during the 1880s, continued almost unabated until the 1950s. The American over the age of thirty-five who still possesses a full set of tonsils and adenoids is a rarity. Yet as early as 1902 reservations about mass tonsillectomies were being raised. In the 1930s medical historian R. F. Packard was still complaining of "the slaughter of tonsils." In 1947 another medical historian, Dr. Arturo Castiglioni, noted that while the popularity of the operation in America has "lessened, the operation still constitutes a mainstay of the specialist's budget."

Infection-fighting drugs like the antibiotics and sulfanilamides made it possible to control tonsil infections without surgery, and so the number of operations performed began to drop. Today the tonsillectomy is a rare operation when compared to the early years of this century, when it seemed that having one's tonsils removed was just another part of growing up.

Were all those operations necessary in the first place? Most medical authorities today think that they were not. Certainly, in cases of severe infection or enlargement, there may have been no other treatment available. But in parts of the world where the operation was not so much in fashion, children did not seem to suffer notably from retaining the troublesome masses of tissue. The tonsils are not just a spare part; they serve a function—to protect against bacterial infection. The casual removal of tonsils may actually have deprived the young patients of just the sort of protection against sore throats the operation was supposed to provide.

Appendectomies, tonsillectomies, gallbladder operations, hysterectomies, and hernia repair are the sort of relatively mundane surgical procedures that most of us either have undergone or will undergo in our lifetimes. But surgery has its heroic, even glamorous, side, and surgeons of unusual skill and daring have become genuine celebrities. There is perhaps no other area of medicine in which the abilities of the individual practitioner are so important. This is particularly true of the surgeons who operate on our two most vital organs, the heart and the brain.

Even before the turn of the century, operations on the heart had been performed successfully. The German surgeon Ludwig Rehn sutured a stab wound of the heart in 1897, and over the next half century hundreds of similar operations were attempted.

In 1938 Robert E. Gross of the Children's Hospital in Boston successfully corrected an open ductus arteriosus in a child aged ten and a half. Open ductus arteriosus is a birth defect that results in blood being shunted away from the heart. Persons born with such a defect had previously been doomed to short and painful lives as cardiac cripples. The operation, which seemed miraculous at the time, became a specialty of Gross's, and it was later adopted by other surgeons.

On the night of May 6, 1958, several million viewers watched the televised heart operation of three-year-old Mabel Chin. The operation to close an open ductus ar-

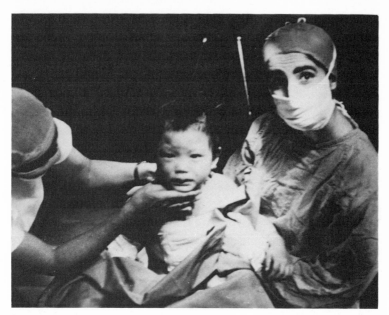

Three-year-old Mabel Chin, whose heart operation was televised in 1958. (New York Heart Association)

teriosus was a success. The televised operation, which had been surrounded with circuslike publicity, had been sponsored by the New York Heart Association in an attempt to dramatize the safety of certain types of heart surgery and to publicize the work of the Heart Association.

But suturing a stab wound to the heart, correcting an open ductus arteriosus, and a few other kinds of operations were relatively easy types of heart surgery because they did not involve stopping the patient's heart. Surgery requiring suspension of heart activity could be carried out only after the development of the heart-lung machine during the 1950s and 1960s. This machine temporarily took over the breathing and the pumping of blood for the heart surgery patient. There was never any single type of heart-lung machine; several different types of machines were developed by different medical teams to carry out the same function. Dr. John H. Gribbon began using a heart-lung machine for open-heart surgery in 1953. The techniques of open-heart surgery have improved steadily, and today thousands of open-heart operations are performed every year. Heart defects are corrected and damaged heart valves replaced, but the most common of all the heart operations is the coronary bypass.

Coronary artery disease is one of the major causes of death in the United States. The arteries leading to the heart become clogged with fatty deposits, blood flow is restricted or stops altogether, and the result is a heart attack and often death. Before the heart itself is actually damaged, however, surgeons are able to replace some of the blocked arteries with arteries taken from the patient's own leg. While no open-heart operation can ever truly be called routine, coronary bypass operations have certainly become common, and the mortality rates for such operations are very low.

Inevitably, the coronary bypass operation also has become clouded by controversy. No one doubts the usefulness of the operation under some circumstances, but critics charge that it is being performed too frequently, and that many heart patients get along just as well with simple changes in diet and life-style. The statistics on whether patients who have had the operation survive longer than patients who have treated their heart conditions without surgery are ambiguous, and so the controversy continues.

The most spectacular of all the heart operations is the complete replacement of a damaged heart with a healthy heart, the heart transplant. Medical scientists had talked about the possibility of such an operation for years, and during the 1960s experiments with animals showed some promise. The successful human heart transplant seemed only a matter of time. When it finally took place, the world, at least the nonmedical world, was amazed and fascinated. The man who first performed this seemingly magical operation was Christiaan Barnard, a forty-five-year-old surgeon at Groote Schuur Hospital in Cape Town, South Africa. The announcement of the operation on December 23, 1967, was flashed as a bulletin across the world. For days Barnard's heart transplant operation was a top news story. Other surgeons who had been preparing to do similar operations may have grumbled a bit when Barnard grabbed the glory of being first.

Barnard's first heart transplant patient died within a few weeks, without ever leaving his hospital bed. A second patient did survive long enough to leave the hospital, though his life outside the hospital was strictly regulated by medical routine.

Soon other surgeons, particularly the Americans Michael De Bakey and Norman Shumway, began performing heart transplants—and the subject remained the top medical news story for several years. It seemed to the layman that a new era had dawned. But the promise of heart transplants had been oversold.

There is no question that the heart transplants were a stunning technical achievement. Less than seventy years earlier a king nearly lost his life because his surgeons had not known how to properly remove his appendix. Now the body's most vital organ could not only be stopped, operated on, and restarted, it could be removed and replaced

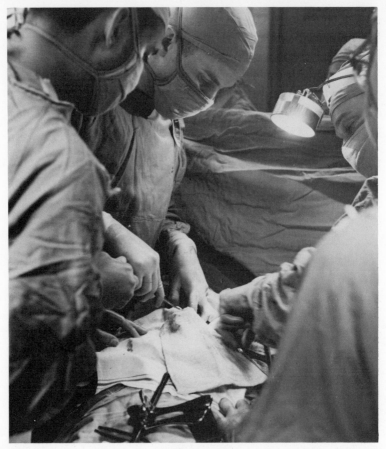

Implanting a pacemaker for the heart. (National Broadcasting Company)

by another. Yet, as even the surgeons performing the operations knew, the heart transplant was not a major surgical procedure and never would be.

The problem of organ rejection had not been solved. When a new heart or any other new organ is transplanted into a body, the body reacts as it does to any other foreign object and does not heal properly. The body's natural defenses against foreign objects must therefore be suppressed by massive doses of drugs, but this leaves the patient open to a host of infections, and besides, the drugs do not always work. It is this rejection rather than any technical deficiency in surgery that kills most heart transplant patients after only a few weeks or months. Kidney transplants are more successful because the kidney is usually donated by a near relative and thus is biologically more compatible with the patient. People have two kidneys and can live quite well with one. But we have only one heart each.

Even if the rejection problem is solved, there will always be a shortage of healthy hearts available for transplantation. There are the very practical considerations that the operation is enormously expensive and time-consuming, and the chances of long-term survival small. Most heart surgeons now feel that their efforts should be directed in more practical and promising channels. The once highly publicized heart transplant is rarely performed today.

If the 1960s had heart surgeons like Barnard and De Bakey as heroes, the early years of the century had its own surgical hero, Harvey Cushing, the surgeon who virtually established the specialty of neurosurgery, or brain surgery.

Since the brain is the most delicate and least understood of human organs, one might imagine that attempts to operate on it are relatively recent. In truth, brain surgery, or at least skull surgery, may be humankind's oldest form of surgery. Skulls from the Neolithic period show that trephining, cutting through the skull to the brain, had been attempted on a surprising number of people in ancient times. Trephining seems to have been practiced in all parts of the world. The operation may have been an attempt to cure severe headaches, or it may have been done for magical reasons, to let the demons or evil spirits out of a person's skull. In at least some of these operations, new growth of bone along the edges of the incisions shows that the individual survived for some time.

While the treatment for headaches had obviously improved by the beginning of the twentieth century, the safety record of brain surgery had not. The mortality rate among those who underwent brain surgery hovered around 90 percent. In the 1920s, when Cushing was at the height of his surgical skill, he had reduced the mortality among his patients to an amazing 8.7 percent.

Cushing did not achieve such a low mortality rate in the most delicate of all forms of surgery through any great medical breakthrough. His success was the result of the painstaking care he took with every procedure in surgery and his almost obsessive desire to learn something new from every operation.

As a young doctor, Cushing had been fortunate to work under Dr. William Halsted of Johns Hopkins medical school. Halsted was a strange and difficult man whose slow and meticulous surgical procedure won both admiration and irritation from his colleagues. He would spend hours on a simple operation that the ordinary surgeon could complete in half the time or less. Halsted tied each blood vessel to keep the operation almost bloodless; he tried to match each wrinkle of the skin when suturing; and he kept his operating room strictly aseptic. There were no postoperative infections in a Halsted operation.

Halsted was also the first to use rubber gloves in surgery, but for a rather unusual reason. His chief nurse, Miss Caroline Hampton, was using an antiseptic that irritated her hands. Halsted was very fond of his nurse; in fact, he later married her. To protect her hands he ordered some rubber gloves for her use. Some of his other aids tried rubber gloves and liked them, and Halsted himself soon saw their advantage in antiseptic surgery. So surgery's most familiar symbol was adopted almost by accident. As one of Halsted's associates put it—"a case where Venus rendered great aid to Aesculapius."

Cushing was, if anything, even more painstaking than his mentor. He was known as a hard taskmaster who lashed out furiously at any of his students or associates who displayed less care and dedication than he did himself. Among his subordinates and colleagues he was not a popular man, but thousands of patients owed their lives to him.

In 1910 Cushing was called upon to treat Major General Leonard Wood. (General Wood had been the commander in Cuba in 1899 during the yellow fever project.) The general had developed a large brain tumor as the result of an injury to his head. Though the tumor was in an area that was extremely difficult to operate on, Cushing nonetheless recommended surgery. The operation took four hours. Eleven days later the general was up and walking around his room. The operation was hailed as a medical miracle, and it made a celebrity out of Harvey Cushing.

Cushing worked like a demon, and in his career he performed well over two thousand brain tumor operations alone. When he gave up the active practice of surgery in 1932, he had plenty of other activities to keep him busy. He became a prolific writer, even winning a Pulitizer Prize for a biography of his friend and associate, the great clinician Sir William Osler. Cushing died in 1939, and an autopsy revealed the supreme irony—he had a brain tumor.

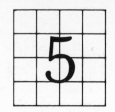

THE PERILS OF WHITE RICE

"Why, you're so bowlegged you can walk over a fire hydrant."

"Did'ja hear the one about the bow-legged fellow and his knock-kneed girlfriend? When they stood together they spelled OX."

There was a lot of that sort of humor at the beginning of the century. The jokes were cruel because no one with grossly deformed legs thought his or her condition was something to laugh about. Yet many had to endure such taunts, because these deformities were common. Most were the result of a disease called rickets, which began in infancy and grew progressively worse through adolescence, when the bones hardened. Rickets was responsible for a variety of other unpleasant symptoms as well, but it was the gross and often grotesque bone deformities that everyone noticed.

Today rickets is virtually unknown in the industrialized world. The nearly total eradication of this bone-deforming disease was not brought about by a new medicine or surgical technique or improvements in sanitation. It was brought about by a few simple changes in diet. Rickets is a nutritional disease—just one of many that have afflicted the human race.

A century ago people didn't know much about the relationship between food and health. There was sort of a general recognition that certain foods "were good for you" and that a varied diet was necessary. But no one quite knew why. Nor was there any general agreement as to what mixture of foods would best promote health. There were plenty of theories, most of which would seem quite bizarre by modern standards.

The great British explorer Captain James Cook insisted that his sailors drink lemon or lime juice during long voyages. This appeared to protect them from a painful and often deadly bleeding disease called scurvy that so often afflicted sailors during long voyages. The British navy adopted Cook's innovation, and the practice incidentally inspired the nickname "limeys" for British seamen. By about 1800 scurvy had virtually ceased to be a problem in the British navy. The lemons and limes worked, though no one had the faintest notion why.

The first real clues to the relationship of what we eat or fail to eat and certain diseases came in 1886 during an investigation of a particularly nasty Oriental disease called beriberi. The word is Sinhalese and means "great weakness," a pretty good description of how those afflicted with the disease feel. The sufferer's arms and legs swell and become crippled by inflammation in the nerves and joints. The heart is affected, and the victim becomes very weak. If the disease progressed, the victim soon died. However, beriberi was not always fatal. Sometimes the stricken would make a nearly miraculous recovery for no known reason. It was a very peculiar disease.

There were all sorts of theories concerning the cause of beriberi, poisoning and poor sanitation among them. But in 1886 the discovery of the germ theory was fresh in the minds of most medical men, and they assumed that beriberi, like so many other diseases, was caused by some sort of microscopic organism.

The Dutch East India Company was having a lot of trouble with beriberi. Many of its soldiers in what was then the Dutch East Indies (now Indonesia) came down with the disease. The Dutch government sent a commission of medical men to the island of Java to find the microbe responsible. It was tough and discouraging work, and after a few months the commission gave up and returned home. But the commission's most tenacious member, Dr. Christiaan Eijkman, stayed behind, convinced that with a bit more work the elusive germ could be isolated and ultimately neutralized.

Then came one of those happy accidents that occur from time to time in scientific research. Perhaps not entirely an accident, for as Louis Pasteur had said, "Chance favors the prepared mind." Eijkman was prepared.

He noticed a group of sick chickens. They wobbled about on swollen legs, their heads hung down at a strange angle—for all the world they looked as if they were suffering from the chicken version of beriberi. Why did this particular flock of chickens succumb to the disease? A few enquiries determined that chickens were not being fed a normal chicken diet. They were being given polished rice, the staple food of the people of the island. Polished rice is rice grain with its fibrous outer hull removed. It is white and tastes better than brown or unpolished rice. When Eijkman put the chickens back on a normal brown rice diet, they recovered almost immediately.

From chickens Eijkman shifted his attention to humans, though not without some resistance from his medical superiors, who thought that he should stop wasting his time on rice and go back to his microscope and look for beriberi germs. Eijkman visited the prisons and found that of 150,000 prisoners fed on polished rich, 400 had beriberi. Of the 96,500 prisoners fed on the cheaper brown rice, only 9 had the disease.

Eijkman made up a brew from the husks of rice and fed it to the sick prisoners. Shortly, all of them recovered.

Simple as it sounds, his conclusion was something truly revolutionary. The men became sick not because of something they had, like a poison or a germ, but because of something they lacked, something contained in the hulls of rice.

Actually, Eijkman was not the first to make this particular observation about beriberi. Six years before Eijkman became interested in sick chickens, a Japanese medical officer named Takaki noticed that sailors who subsisted on a straight white rice diet often came down with beriberi, while sailors who were able to supplement their diets with meat, vegetables, and barley almost never did. Takaki thought the disease was caused by something missing in the diet; he suggested protein. That suggestion was wrong, but his basic idea was absolutely correct. However, Takaki's insights were ignored, and so very nearly were Eijkman's, because most medical researchers were still looking for the nonexistent beriberi germ.

Eijkman was unable to isolate the exact element in rice hulls that prevented beriberi. That didn't help his case either. But there was no doubt that he had figured out a method of protecting people from beriberi. When half the prison population of Java was put on brown rice, they complained bitterly, but not a single one of these prisoners developed the disease. Among the "lucky" prisoners who still had the luxury of eating the tastier polished rice, it was beriberi as usual.

In 1912 a Cambridge University biochemist named Frederick Gowland Hopkins first demonstrated the existence of what he called "accessory food substances" in a series of carefully controlled experiments with rats. These food substances were accessory to the main food groups such as fats and carbohydrates, which were already known. Later that year the Polish-born chemist Casimir Funk coined the term *vitamines* (later changed to vitamins) to describe these substances. Funk said that he wanted a descriptive phrase that would also make a good catchword. He certainly got that.

In Funk's opinion not only beriberi but scurvy, rickets, and pellagra were caused by a lack of certain vitamins in the diet. Pellagra was a disease common among poor people in the rural South. In the mildest form of pellagra, the symptom was only a reddish and roughened skin, a bit like a sunburn. This could progress rapidly to severe sores on the skin and headaches. The disease also affected the mind; the sufferer would become nervous, depressed, apathetic, and confused. As the disease became worse, those afflicted would begin to have hallucinations and become completely disoriented. Untreated, the result was total insanity and inevitably death. The mental suffering of the pellagra victim could become so great that death was a welcome relief. Pellagra was a terrifying disease.

During the early years of this century, pellagra was

making alarming headway in the southern states. In a single year the state of Mississippi alone recorded more than fifteen hundred deaths from the disease. The story of the discovery of the cause and cure of this once common scourge contains one of those truly inspiring accounts of medical heroism.

The hero was Dr. Joseph Goldberger, who had been sent to Mississippi early in 1914 to investigate pellagra for the U.S. Public Health Service. Dr. Goldberger had already done work on typhus and yellow fever, both infectious diseases. At first glance pellagra appeared to be a similar type of affliction. It was almost exclusively a disease of the poor, those who lived in crowded cabins without any running water or toilets. The general assumption was that pellagra was caused by some sort of microbe and was spread by unsanitary living conditions.

But as Goldberger began to observe the progress of the disease more closely, he found that the pattern of its spread was different from what might be expected if it was

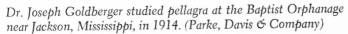

Dr. Joseph Goldberger studied pellagra at the Baptist Orphanage near Jackson, Mississippi, in 1914. (Parke, Davis & Company)

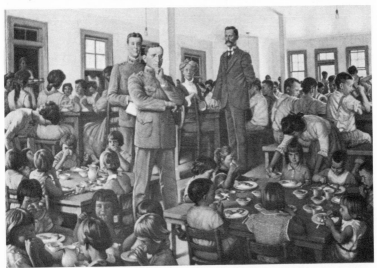

an ordinary infectious disease. In hospitals where pellagra victims were taken, doctors and nurses never seemed to "catch" it, though they certainly would have been thoroughly exposed to any germs. In prisons many of the inmates contracted the disease, the guards never did.

Goldberger quickly became convinced that the difference between those who got the disease and those who seemed immune to it was diet. In 1914 the southern poor lived on diets made up mostly of cornmeal mush, hominy grits, and cane syrup, with an occasional piece of salt pork. The better off, who did not get the disease, supplemented their diets with meat, milk, and fresh vegetables.

Goldberger suspected a nutritional cause for the disease, but he had to prove it to a medical world still looking for germs. The first step was an experiment with eleven convict volunteers. They were placed on a diet of mush, molasses, grits, cabbage, potatoes, and rice—just the sort of diet that was quite familiar to poor pellagra victims. The other living conditions of the convicts were improved. Yet within five months all eleven showed the telltale reddish and rough skin that marked the first stages of the disease.

That strengthened the case for a nutritional link but did not prove it conclusively. The next step was to prove pellagra wasn't a bacteria-caused, communicable disease. Goldberger took samples of blood, urine, feces, and peeling skin of pellagra victims and injected them into a group of volunteers. He was the first volunteer, his wife the second, and all of the other volunteers in this potentially dangerous experiment were Goldberger's medical associates. No one in the group suffered anything worse than a sore arm. Goldberger had shown, in the most dramatic way possible, that he had confidence in his theory and in the safety of the experiment he was conducting.

The exact substance or vitamin that protected against pellagra was unknown to Dr. Goldberger (some years later the missing vitamin, B_2, was identified). But after a series of experiments, and a lucky accident, he discovered a cheap and easy method for preventing the disease. Simply adding a small amount of common brewer's yeast to the diet provided absolute protection against pellagra.

A diet deficient in vitamin D is the cause of rickets. That vitamin proved to be unusually difficult to locate, and long before it was, the most popular preventative was oil taken from the liver of a cod fish. For a large part of the twentieth century, children all over the world reluctantly swallowed daily doses of the smelly, fishy oil. Nasty tasting as it was, it was a very small price to pay for prevention of the bone-deforming disease.

After their existence was established, vitamins did not remain mysterious substances for long. Laboratories got to work on them. One by one, more than thirty vitamins were identified, isolated, and synthesized. The world, and most particularly the United States, began to go a little vitamin crazy.

Vitamins, as it turned out, were not the only indispensable nutrients. "In 1900," one of the nutrition pioneers has written, "we were almost blind to the relations of food to health." But nutrition research over the next two decades showed very clearly that the connection between proper nutrition and good health was profound but very complex. First came the discovery of the vitamins. Successive studies revealed the need for minute amounts of amino acids and minerals in the healthy diet.

The impact the discovery of vitamins and other nutrients had on most people's thinking about health is difficult to overestimate. Here were simple, cheap, substances that could be administered in a tasty, or at least not too unpleasant, manner, and they could prevent or cure some of the worst diseases. What else could vitamins and other nutrients do?

That question cannot be fully answered even today. Starting in the 1920s, a huge variety of vitamin pills, extracts, compounds, and vitamin-enriched foods began flooding the market. Some of the claims made for these products rivaled the claims made for the old-fashioned patent medicines.

As the number of "wonder vitamin" products grew, so did opposition to them from the orthodox medical community and ultimately from government agencies, primarily the Food and Drug Administration. Most scientists insisted that health could be maintained through eating a well-balanced diet—no vitamin supplements of any kind were needed under normal conditions. But what were normal conditions? Besides, surveys had shown that during the 1930s, even in the United States, as many as one-third of the nation's families were not eating a well-balanced or even adequate diet.

Finally, scientists tried to make some order out of the nutritional chaos. In 1940 the National Academy of Sciences and the National Research Council set up a Food and Nutrition Board that was to develop a list of "Recommended Daily Allowances for Specific Nutrients." In 1941 the first list was issued, indicating the number of calories and the quantities of nine nutrients needed for good nutrition by an average healthy person. The board acknowledged that people who were sick or already suffering from some kind of malnutrition might need more of a specific nutrient than the list indicated. The board also admitted the limits of scientific knowledge on the subject by pointing out that there were at least eleven other known nutrients for which no recommended daily allowances could be established because of inadequate data.

In view of the fact that surveys had shown an alarming percentage of the nation's population to be inadequately nourished, the board recommended that some foods be "enriched" with vitamins that had been synthesized in the laboratory. This was not the first time foods were enriched for health reasons. Goiter, a disfiguring enlargement of the thyroid gland in the front of the neck, had once been a common condition in the United States. The condition is caused by a deficiency of iodine in the diet, and as early as 1924 iodine had been added to salt to prevent the development of goiter. Vitamin D had been added to milk and vitamin A to margarine. The Food and Nutrition Board also proposed enriching bread and other grain products with several different vitamins and iron. All of these recommendations were carried out.

Some of today's breakfast foods boast that a single serving contains all the vitamins you need for the day. That sort of claim is not new, and many of today's most popular breakfast foods started originally as health foods. In Battle Creek, Michigan, center for early-twentieth-century breakfast cereal manufacture, there existed a curious mixture of health, religion, and business. Corn Flakes were first known as "Elija's Manna," and Grape Nuts were suggested as a preventative for appendicitis.

When the United States entered World War II, the nation was afflicted with a variety of food shortages. Yet because nutritional standards had already been established, the sort of outbreaks of disease that had previously accompanied food shortages did not occur. This general rise in the nation's nutritional standards is one of the most significant health advances of the last century. Because it lacks the drama of the discovery of a new vaccine or the perfection of some new and heroic form of surgery, it is not a well-known area of medical history.

While the list of minimum daily requirements of nutrients has grown and changed since 1941, it is still with us. You can find a listing printed on the boxes of breakfast cereals and other foods. Most authorities continue to insist that for normally healthy individuals who eat a balanced diet no vitamin supplements are necessary. And yet the vitamin industry is now a multibillion-dollar business in the United States. Most drugstores and supermarkets have large displays of an astounding variety of vitamins and/or minerals, all of which are for sale without a prescription. Perhaps you regularly take one of these "unnecessary" vitamin supplements yourself. Most people do at one time or another. Despite what orthodox medical authorities insist, millions of Americans believe that additional vitamins will help them get healthy or remain healthy in some unspecified way. At the very least, the vitamins couldn't hurt.

During the 1920s and early 1930s some of the multivitamin and mineral promoters advertised their products as cures or preventatives for a host of specific ailments such as high blood pressure and even cancer. Such claims quickly ran afoul of laws regulating medical advertising. Vitamin and mineral advertisers then switched to less specific claims such as saying that their particular product was good for "tired blood"—an effective-sounding but utterly meaningless phrase. Supplements and tonics promised to "increase vigor" or "prevent wearing out" because of nutritional deficiency. Even such vague claims were often contested by the government. Currently, most over-the-counter vitamin advertising makes no claims at all. Advertisements for one of the most popular compounds shows healthy-looking older people who say that they "take care" of themselves by taking one tablet daily. This very general sales pitch appears to work very well.

While the majority of today's physicians do not believe that massive doses of vitamins can cure or alleviate any of the serious ailments for which there is no known cure, there are a minority of perfectly respectable physicians who use so-called megavitamin therapy in treating a whole host of ailments, including some forms of mental illness. And they claim remarkable success, though such success has been hard to document.

The biggest vitamin and health controversy of the last twenty years was touched off by Linus Pauling, a Nobel Prize-winning biochemist and a man generally recognized as one of the most brilliant and innovative scientists of the twentieth century. Pauling announced that in his opinion massive doses of vitamin C, far in excess of the "minimum daily requirements," would help prevent the common cold or temper the severity of a cold. Such a statement simply flew in the face of conventional thinking about the uses of vitamins. Most medical authorities politely brushed the suggestion aside—one does not denounce a man of Pauling's stature. But the publicity surrounding the Pauling theory sent millions rushing to the drugstore for bottles of vitamin C. So great was the rush that for months drugstores throughout the country were unable to keep vitamin C in stock. Today it is still the country's best-selling vitamin.

A number of attempts have been made to test the Pauling theory of vitamin C and colds. The results of these tests have been contradictory and ambiguous. It is far harder to test the efficiency of most treatments or preventatives than the general public imagines. Pauling has stuck to his theory, and millions continue to take their daily doses of vitamin C, in the belief or hope that it will protect them from the common cold.

In the first part of the last hundred years, medical concern was centered on what was left out of diets. In recent decades, concern has switched to what is being put in. The last forty years have seen a major revolution in the ways in which food is grown, prepared, and preserved. What has happened in food production is really just part of the broader chemical revolution, which has reached into all parts of our lives. Such substances as antibiotics used to help fatten cattle and certain preservatives and food colorings have been withdrawn or their use sharply reduced because there is evidence that they can be harmful.

The public has shown a good deal of anxiety over the safety of a broad range of chemicals used in food production. There has been an unprecedented boom in the sales of "natural" foods, that is, foods that are grown and marketed without adding any "chemicals."

As with vitamins, the bulk of the medical profession has taken a conservative stand toward these fears. The general attitude is that today's foods are safer and more nutritious than they have ever been. These assurances are not necessarily believed, and a lot of people still worry about "chemical additives" and seek out "natural" foods even if they are more expensive.

The relationship between nutrition and health has developed into one of the most controversial areas for modern medical science to deal with. It is likely to remain so for a long time to come.

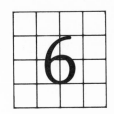

PUBLIC HEALTH AND PREVENTIVE MEDICINE

CHOLERA WAS A terrible disease that regularly ravaged London and other cities during the nineteenth century. One of the worst outbreaks ever took place in Broad Street in London in 1854. In a small area there were more than five hundred fatal cases in ten days.

At the time, no one knew what caused cholera, but the physician John Snow suspected that whatever the cause, the disease was spread by water taken from a popular street pump in Broad Street. Snow questioned people in the area of the outbreak and found that virtually everyone who came down with the disease drank water taken from the pump. Broad Street brewery workers rarely got cholera because they had a beer allowance and didn't drink much water. Snow had the handle of the Broad Street pump removed—and the cholera epidemic in Broad Street ended, as if by magic.

Snow's investigation of the Broad Street pump is

regarded as one of the classics of early epidemiology. His solution to the deadly problem of cholera was extremely simple and effective.

During the nineteenth century, medical authorities realized that people needed clean drinking water, good drainage, and adequate removal of rubbish if many diseases were to be held in check. This was true even if the exact cause of the disease remained unknown. These simple principles seem obvious to us today, yet they were not during the nineteenth century. There was all manner of resistance to sanitary measures. People did not always see the relationship between filth and disease, since few cases were as clear as that of the Broad Street pump. Even Snow's findings were not generally accepted at first. No medical journal would publish them, and he had to bring them out at his own expense.

People had always dumped their garbage into the streets or the river. They didn't like being told they couldn't do it anymore. Disease—well, that was just one of God's afflictions and had to be borne.

The greatest objections to sanitation were economic. It cost money to clean up the filth. Besides, those who suffered the worst from unsanitary conditions were generally the poor and the powerless, though no one was immune. Prince Albert, Queen Victoria's consort, died of typhoid, a disease that is completely controllable by proper sanitary measures. It often took a disaster like the cholera epidemic in Broad Street to have changes put into effect. The establishment of the rules of proper sanitation has probably saved more lives than all the drugs and other medical advances of the nineteenth century. It stopped the diseases before they got started. Prevention is always the best medicine.

By the end of the nineteenth century, the need for proper sanitation was finally established, and despite occasional foot dragging by cost-conscious authorities or by people who were just plain ignorant, cities and towns were being cleaned up.

Thus, the major steps in the sanitary control of infectious diseases took place more than a century ago. However, public health problems are far from solved, for during the last hundred years the focus has shifted to a whole new set of medical problems. Many of the century-old arguments about sanitation are being replayed, with only the names of the diseases changed.

Let's start with the health effects of air pollution. Of course, people have been complaining about smoky, dirty air for centuries, just as they had complained about open sewers for hundreds of years before anything was done about them. The relationship between dirty air and disease was difficult to establish, and even more difficult to get people concerned about. The word *smog* was first coined way back in 1905 by a London physician, Dr. Harold Des Voeux, one of the most prominent leaders in the fight for smoke control. Yet this very evocative word did not come into common usage for fifty years, and then it came by way of California.

Back in 1905 there was very little worry about air pollution, or smog or whatever you wanted to call it, outside the ranks of a few crusaders like Dr. Des Voeux. Such crusaders were considered a bit eccentric, even a bit fanatical. The badly polluted London air had almost been given a romantic quality. This is how a bad London smog was described by the physician-writer Arthur Conan Doyle in the Sherlock Holmes story *The Bruce Partington Plans*:

In the third week of November in the year 1895, a dense yellow fog settled down upon London. From the Monday to the Thursday I doubt whether it was ever possible from our windows in Baker Street to see the loom of the opposite houses. The first day Holmes had spent in cross-indexing his huge book of references. The second and third had been patiently occupied upon a subject which he had recently made his hobby —the music of the Middle Ages. But when, for the fourth time, after pushing back our chairs from breakfast we saw the greasy, heavy brown swirl still drifting past us and condensing in oily drops upon the window-panes, my comrade's impatient and active nature could endure this drab existence no longer.

A short time later Holmes remarks, " 'Look out of this window, Watson. See how the figures loom up, are dimly seen, and then blend once more into the cloud-bank. The thief or the murderer could roam London on such a day as the tiger does the jungle, unseen until he pounces, and then evident only to his victim.' "

The "greasy, heavy brown swirl" did more than provide cover for criminals. It irritated the eyes and throat and made people cough and wheeze, though Conan Doyle did not mention this. Few thought that the "yellow fog" might have serious long-term effects or that the effects would be serious enough to warrant making any major changes in the way Londoners lived and worked. No one but a smoke-abatement fanatic would have thought the fog deadly. Yet it was a greater killer than any Sherlock Holmes ever faced.

The smoke that turned the fog to smog came from the great industrial plants of London and from thousands upon thousands of smoky coal fires in private homes. Businessmen scorned the feeble efforts of clean-air reformers;

indeed they almost prided themselves on the amount of smoke their factories produced. A smoky chimney was a sign of a thriving industry. "Muck is money" was a slogan of the time. The average London householder loved his coal fire with its cheery glow. Besides, there was plenty of soft coal in England, and a coal fire was the cheapest way to stay warm. Smarting eyes and a hacking cough for a few days a year seemed a small price to pay.

There were some statistical indications that during periods of extremely severe air pollution the death rate rose, particularly among the elderly or those who suffered from chronic heart or respiratory diseases. Still, few connected this rising death rate with the air itself.

On December 1, 1930, a mass of stagnant, foggy air settled over the heavily industrialized Meuse valley in Belgium. Though the air had become dark and acrid, the industries of the valley continued to pump a variety of pollutants into the atmosphere. After three days the people of the valley began to feel sick, and some of them died. The smog lasted six days, and before it had dispersed, several hundred people had become seriously ill and some sixty had died.

Amazingly, at first very few people suspected what had happened. There were rumors of mysterious airplanes dropping poison gas on the valley, of an industrial accident with lethal fumes leaking out of a broken pipe, even of an outbreak of bubonic plague. An investigation proved it was none of these things, that the cause of the illnesses and deaths was the smoke that issued daily from the factories of the valley.

Near the end of October 1948 there was another major air pollution disaster, this one in the United States. It centered in the industrial town of Donora, Pennsylvania, about thirty miles south of Pittsburgh. The causes of the disaster were much the same as they had been in the Meuse valley: stagnant air that trapped the smoke from the town's many factories. The smog lasted four days before it was washed away by a rain. It took approximately seventeen lives, and an estimated 40 percent of the town's ten thousand inhabitants had been made ill.

This time the U.S. Public Health Service conducted a thorough investigation of the Donora tragedy. The unavoidable conclusion was that air pollution, and air pollution alone, was responsible for what happened. The report on Donora was given wide circulation, and for the first time large numbers of people began to realize that air pollution could be a serious, even deadly problem. Very little was done to avert future possible air pollution tragedies, however.

Just a month after the Donora disaster, there was a major smog episode in London that killed an estimated three hundred people, mostly elderly or ill. This event attracted little attention, for the official and unofficial attitude of British government and industry seems to have been that the premature death of a small number of individuals who were "hanging on the edge" was the inevitable price one had to pay for the comforts, convenience, and profits of modern life. It was what might be called an economic trade-off. Of course, few in public life could express these opinions quite so boldly, but that's what it came down to.

Finally, there came a smog disaster in London that simply could not be shrugged off as an unfortunate but necessary part of life. It began on December 4, 1952. Cold still air had settled over the city, and a temperature inversion developed. The air at the surface became colder and was trapped by a layer of warmer air above. There was little or no air movement upward or laterally, thus smoke, soot, and anything else that was pumped into the atmosphere stayed there. These conditions remained virtually unchanged for four days and four nights. The color of the smog went from white, to yellow, to amber, to black, as factories, power stations, trucks, buses, and thousands of domestic chimneys continued to pour smoke into the air.

During the period of the fog, all most people talked about was how dark it had become. The coughing and burning eyes were taken as a normal part of life. It took quite a while for people to realize that something quite terrible had happened. For the first few days after the fog lifted, the newspapers reported only that there had been an increase in traffic accidents and crime, and that a large number of meetings and other events had to be canceled because of the premature darkness. A week or more passed before the outlines of the tragedy became known, and then they came out in bits and pieces. The newspapers began to run stories of overcrowding in hospitals, and of "one of the worst funeral holdups since the 1918 flu epidemic." By the middle of December the *British Medical Journal* estimated that the smog had been responsible for the deaths of nearly 5,000 Londoners. It was worse than the worst nineteenth-century outbreak of cholera. In addition to the deaths, there were between 50,000 and 100,000 serious illnesses that resulted from breathing the polluted air during the four days of the killer smog. The long-term effects of this episode have never been determined. However, in the light of today's knowledge of air pollution we can assume that the smog contributed to the development of such diseases as bronchitis, emphysema, and lung cancer in a large number of individuals.

At first some authorities groped about looking for a

new germ that had caused the "mysterious fog illness." There was nothing at all mysterious about what had happened. According to a medical report issued two months after the disaster:

". . . The London fog of December 1952 was no strange new phenomenon. It was no acute epidemic caused by a hitherto unrecognized virus nor was it a visitation of some known pathogen against which we had no defense. It was simply the occurrence of a well-known meteorological phenomenon in an area where the toxic products of combustion are vomited in excess into the air. . . ."

Disasters such as the one in London in 1952 finally awakened the general public to the dangers of air pollution, and the governments of Britain, the United States, and a few other countries slowly and often reluctantly began to pass a variety of laws aimed at cleaning up the air.

As the story of the Broad Street pump shows, the dangers of some forms of water pollution were recognized well over a hundred years ago. Yet until recently only one type of contaminated water has been treated as a serious problem, water contamination by bacteria. Over the last hundred years public health measures have been very successful in controlling epidemics of once dangerous waterborne diseases like cholera.

By the middle of the twentieth century it was commonly believed that the major water supplies in the advanced, industrialized nations of the world were entirely safe to drink. We can no longer be sure that this is true, for a new menace has developed and been recognized. It is the pollution of water with toxic chemical wastes. While techniques for ridding water of bacterial wastes are well known, getting rid of chemical wastes is not nearly as easy.

We don't even know how great the health problem posed by these wastes really is.

During the past fifty years or so there has been an enormous expansion in the chemical industry. Thousands upon thousands of new chemicals have been produced. The wastes from production and use of these chemicals have often been dumped into rivers, streams, lakes, and sometimes the ocean. Some of these wastes have been stored on land in drums. As over the years these drums have corroded, the chemical wastes have seeped into the ground and eventually turned up in wells and other water supply sources.

When the chemical revolution in industry really got rolling in the United States in the years after World War II, no one thought much about the possible health hazards of chemical wastes. Naturally, no one was allowed to pour known poisons into the water supply. But so much was unknown. There were virtually no restrictions about dumping most chemicals. Chemical wastes were, after all, not bacteria. Such wastes rarely produced instant illness like cholera, or the acute and obvious respiratory symptoms that can be seen during episodes of severe air pollution. The concentrations of toxic wastes in water are generally small, and the ill effects, if any, build up over a period of many years. A direct causal relationship between toxic wastes in water and cancer, kidney disease, birth defects, or any other conditions that may develop slowly over ten or twenty years, is difficult to establish. Yet no one seriously doubts that such a relationship can exist. The problem is complicated by the fact that there usually are several different chemicals in the water, and the effects of a mixture of chemicals is unknown.

In the United States, awareness of the potential

problem grew during the 1970s. The Love Canal, a badly polluted area near the city of Buffalo, New York, became a symbol for the nation and the world. For many years the Hooker Chemical Company had used the canal as a site for dumping chemical wastes, many of them poisonous or cancer producing. The Love Canal area became so saturated with these wastes that residents not only were unable to drink the water, they had to abandon their homes. Hooker claimed that it was not responsible for the damages because it had been acting in accordance with established practices at the time. Besides, the chemical company claimed, the dangers had been grossly exaggerated, and the near hysteria that had developed among Love Canal residents was excessive and unnecessary.

Many once prosperous fishing and shellfishing areas have been closed because the catch taken from them was found to contain high concentrations of dangerous chemicals. Wells and other public water supplies once thought to be completely safe were found to be badly polluted by dangerous chemicals. Often they were also closed.

The health problems posed by water and air pollution are solvable. Great strides toward overcoming them, particularly in the area of air pollution, were made during the 1960s and 1970s. The air in many of the major cities in the United States and throughout much of Europe improved markedly through the enforcement of a variety of clean-air regulations, which affected everything from the burning of garbage to automobile emissions. The progress against water pollution by toxic chemicals was slower. But even there, tough regulations forced many industries to handle potentially dangerous chemical wastes with greater care.

None of this progress came cheaply. There is a price tag, often a big one, attached to cleaner air and cleaner water. The question of how much our society is willing to pay is a political as well as a medical one. Some people say the cost is too high, there are too many government regulations, and the problem isn't as bad as all that anyway. The battles that one hundred years or more ago were being fought over open sewers and garbage in the streets are now being refought over the newer problems of chemical pollution.

Another area of public health concern is industrial safety. One hundred years ago the average industrial worker had practically no protection on the job, but that has changed today. Dangerous machines have been made safer, and mines and other hazardous workplaces are inspected regularly. Workers on certain types of jobs are given goggles to protect their eyes or hard hats to protect their heads.

Machines that can chew up hands and arms and gas-filled mines are the obvious hazards in the workplace. There are less obvious hazards, and these have been more difficult to correct successfully. The potential dangers of a coal mine explosion are well known, and to a certain extent can be guarded against. But many miners develop a debilitating condition known as black lung. It is caused by years of breathing air laced with coal dust. Coal mining has been going on for centuries, and for centuries miners have been made invalids or had their lives shortened by black lung. Yet this very serious medical condition was barely even acknowledged until the 1950s.

Asbestos, a very effective fire retardant, was widely used in industry and construction. It was particularly useful in shipbuilding, for shipboard fires are one of the great dangers of the sea. During the shipbuilding boom of World War II, thousands upon thousands of American shipyard workers were exposed to enormous concentrations of asbestos dust. The asbestos was often sprayed onto parts of the ship, and no one thought twice about breathing in the clouds of white powder that filled the air. It made the nose and throat itch, that seemed to be all. It wasn't.

Twenty years later epidemiologists found that an alarming percentage of shipyard workers developed a rare and exceptionally lethal form of lung cancer. The cause of the disease was the asbestos particles that lodged in the workers' lungs. Even the families of shipyard workers were not safe. A man would come home from work, his clothes covered with asbestos fibers. His wife would shake out the overalls, sometimes in the yard where the children were playing. Twenty years later the entire family would be stricken with asbestos-created cancer.

Today the dangers of breathing in asbestos fibers are well known. The dangers are so well know that a 1979 government report indicating that certain brands of hair driers contained asbestos set off a near panic, though the danger from such driers was slight. During the 1940s, when all the ships were being built, no one knew or even suspected that this very useful and innocent-looking material would turn out to be a killer.

How many other potential workplace dangers are out there, particularly in this era when thousands upon thousands of new materials have been introduced? The truth is that no one really knows.

Not only have the air and water come under scrutiny but the medical effects of our personal habits have also

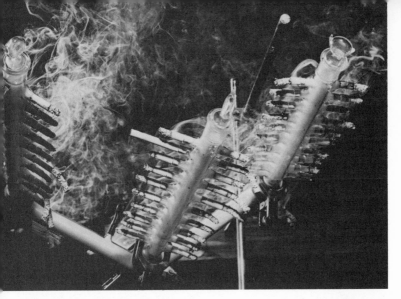

A *smoking machine used in the investigation of cigarette smoking.*
(American Cancer Society)

been an issue during the last one hundred years. Take, for example, smoking. From the time that tobacco was first introduced, there have been those who objected to it as a "filthy habit." Smoking, particularly cigarette smoking, always carried with it a faint air of immorality. During the early years of the twentieth century, it was considered shocking for women to smoke, particularly in public. Cigarette advertisers worked hard and successfully to change that image. Youngsters were told that smoking would "stunt their growth" or have some other vague bad effects upon their health. Such objections were based primarily on old wives' tales. Hard evidence of the medical dangers of smoking didn't really begin to appear until the 1950s.

Once again, the problem in spotting the dangers was that the illnesses were slow in coming. Smokers didn't suddenly come down with something. The diseases related to smoking, lung cancer, emphysema, heart disease, and bronchitis, develop gradually, and not every smoker succumbs. It was only after massive statistical studies were

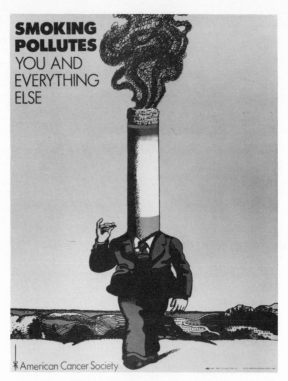

Poster for an anti-smoking campaign. (American Cancer Society)

carried on over a period of many years that the close relationship of these diseases to smoking was revealed.

Government health authorities in Britain were the
first to strongly denounce smoking. Later the surgeon general of the United States issued similar warnings. The sale
and advertising of cigarettes was restricted. There were
private and government-sponsored campaigns against smoking, but the sale of tobacco was not banned. Such a ban
would probably never have worked, because for many people
smoking is a deeply ingrained habit, perhaps even an addiction. Prohibition had never stopped people from drinking.

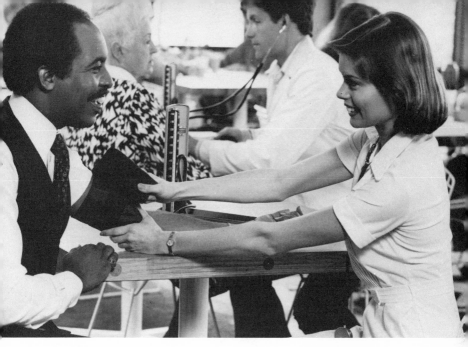

Mass screening for high blood pressure is one of the methods used to identify potential heart disease victims. (American Heart Association)

Tobacco manufacturers continue to claim that no direct causal relationship between smoking and lung cancer or other diseases has been established. No direct causal relationship between cholera and the Broad Street pump had been established in 1854 either. But when people stopped using the pump they stopped getting cholera. Medical authorities are practically unanimous in asserting that smoking contributes mightily to a host of serious diseases, including the two leading killers, heart disease and cancer. They also assert that giving up smoking, or avoiding it in the first place, is the single best thing that anyone can do for his or her health.

The public in general has been convinced that smoking is bad for health, but it's an easy habit to get into and a tough one to break, particularly since the painful consequences may be delayed many, many years. While the campaigns against smoking have been successful in reducing the number of people who smoke and have probably prevented many from starting, smoking still remains a major health problem, some people think *the* major preventable health problem, in many parts of the world.

Heart disease and associated circulatory diseases remain the number-one killers in the United States and most industrialized nations of the world. As with cancer, the exact causes of these diseases are not known. But it is suspected that our dietary and personal habits, including smoking, contribute to these diseases.

We have been urged to eat less and cut down particularly on certain types of fatty foods, and to exercise more. One hundred years ago, those who could afford them ate gargantuan meals of rich foods and exercised as little as possible. Few thought they might be damaging their health. Plumpness was considered a sign of financial and physical well-being. It's hard to imagine what a fellow like William Howard Taft, our three-hundred-pound president and later Supreme Court chief justice, would have thought of a low-cholesterol diet and jogging.

During the 1970s the high rates of death from heart disease in the United States, which had been rising for nearly a century, began to fall for the first time. The reasons for this reduction are not altogether clear, but most medical authorities believe that certain changes in personal habits, such as avoidance of cigarettes, weight reduction, low-fat diets, and increased exercise, are the primary reasons for the change. They are far more important than any new medical treatment or drugs.

As always, preventive medicine is the best medicine.

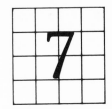

THE CHEMICAL REVOLUTION

THE STANDARD COMPLAINT about the modern doctor is that if you call him at night, no matter what your symptoms he will tell you, "Take two aspirins and call me in the morning."

A century ago the doctor might have come to your house. But he couldn't have told you to take two aspirins because that most ubiquitous of today's remedies hadn't been invented yet.

Aspirin has a rather curious history. It began back in the early days of antiseptic surgery. The English surgeon Joseph Lister insisted that carbolic acid be used freely in the operating room to wash the instruments and to spray in a patient's wounds. The washes and sprays did help to reduce the dangers of infection drastically, but carbolic acid was irritating and evil smelling. It was also highly poisonous and thus could not be used to prevent internal infections.

99

A German chemist named Hermann Kolbe suggested the use of salicylic acid, chemically similar to carbolic acid but nonpoisonous. Salicylic acid became the wonder drug of its day, at first. Not only could it be used in place of the reeking carbolic but when patients swallowed it they felt better.

It took about a year for doctors to realize that patients who swallowed salicylic acid died from typhoid, pneumonia, or other infections at the same rate as patients who didn't take it. The substance was not an internal infection fighter, it didn't kill germs, but it did make people feel better temporarily by reducing fever and deadening pain. Salicylic acid wasn't supposed to reduce fever or kill pain, and no one knew why it worked, but it was cheaper than quinine, the favored fever reducer of the day, and safer than morphine, the most popular painkiller. It was Dr. Carl Emil Buss who first made this observation. Buss's discovery was greeted with great enthusiasm by doctors around the world, who immediately began using the substance.

In 1883 another German chemist, Ludwig Knorr, put together a compound called antipyrine. Like salicylic acid, antipyrine reduced fevers and deadened pain. It was also the first important completely man-made drug, and its invention launched a spectacular new industry—the synthetic drug business.

Antipyrine was not only successful at reducing fevers and deadening pain, it was also a huge money-maker, and its success inspired practically every industrial chemist in Germany to try to find an even more profitable rival. The prize ultimately went to Felix Hoffman, a chemist at the giant Friedrich Bayer dye works. Hoffman determined to test every known compound of salicylic acid for its pain-killing and fever-reducing properties. In the chemical literature he read of the production, years before, of a derivative of salicylic acid called acetylsalicylic acid. At the time, the product had been regarded as a chemical oddity, with little practical use. The name of acetylsalicylic acid's discoverer had long been forgotten. Hoffman turned the compound over to the Bayer medical department for testing. The results were spectacular—this substance was by far the most effective yet mildest painkiller and fever reducer yet known. Once on the market it would make a fortune.

But there was the problem of the name. Acetylsalicylic acid was cumbersome. While the chemical itself had been produced synthetically since 1856, it did occur in nature in the oil of the spiraea leaf. Acetylspiraea was shortened to acetylspirin and finally to aspirin.

Aspirin is nearly a century old, and it is still the most widely used drug in the world.

While the synthetic drug industry really began with the discovery of aspirin and like substances around the turn of the century, the rush of new drugs onto the market did not begin for several decades. A case in point is the important infection-fighting drug sulfanilamide. The basic compound was first produced in 1908 by a German scientist named Gelmo, and it was rediscovered in later years by several other scientists. But its properties as an infection fighter were not recognized until 1932. Even then, use of the drug was held up for several years because of a business dispute. The crucial experiments had been conducted in the laboratories of the giant I. G. Farben chemical company in Germany. However, Farben executives delayed public announcement of the life-saving discovery while they attempted to obtain worldwide patent rights. People who could have been saved by sulfanilamide were dying while Farben delayed. Word of the discovery leaked out, and other scientists began experimenting with similar compounds. In 1935 French investigators were not only able to reproduce the German discovery, they had improved on it. The final product could be cheaply and easily produced. Sulfanilamide was not the universal germ killer that some scientists first hoped it might be. But it was better than anything else around.

Use of the new drug in the United States got an enormous boost in November 1936. Franklin Roosevelt, Jr., the president's son, contracted a serious and dangerous streptococcus infection of the throat. The president's wife, Eleanor, telephoned Drs. P. H. Long and E. A. Bliss of Johns Hopkins University in Baltimore. Long and Bliss were conducting tests with the new drug. Eleanor Roosevelt had heard of the tests, and she asked if the drug might be used on her son. Long went to Washington and administered sulfanilamide to young Roosevelt, who was soon out of danger and well on his way to recovery.

The successful treatment of the president's son received national press attention, and quite suddenly doctors all over the country began showing an interest in sulfanilamide. Previously, physician and patient acceptance of radical new treatments like sulfanilamide was slow in coming, but that attitude was changing. Laboratories were hard at work fabricating new varieties of the drug. Soon there was a whole family of infection-fighting sulfa drugs available.

When the United States entered World War II, the armed forces medical departments were well supplied with these new drugs, and the sulfa drugs were credited with saving many thousands of soldiers and civilians who would otherwise have perished from blood poisoning and other infections.

Every American soldier carried a packet of sulfa drugs in his kit. When wounded, he was to sprinkle some of the powdered drug into the wound to prevent infection. The drug was often effective enough in holding off infection to allow time for the wounded man to be taken to a hospital behind the lines, rather than having a hasty operation or other treatment performed under battlefield conditions. In past wars any serious wound was commonly a death sentence, for if the wound itself did not prove fatal, the inevitable infection did. Military hospitals were often just places where the wounded were taken to die, or, if they were lucky, to have an arm or leg amputated. With the introduction of the sulfa drugs this grim picture was altered.

Sulfa drugs were not perfect. They could produce unpleasant, even dangerous, side effects. The body quickly built up a tolerance to them, and higher and higher doses were needed. Most tellingly, they simply were not effective in many cases. Ironically, a far more effective infection-fighting agent had already been discovered, and was languishing for lack of attention.

This, of course, was penicillin. There has perhaps never been a more apt demonstration of Louis Pasteur's dictum that chance favors the prepared mind than the story of Alexander Fleming's discovery of penicillin. In 1928 Fleming was an obscure teacher and researcher at Saint Mary's Hospital in London. For years he had been working on various types of antiseptics. As part of his work he grew bacteria cultures in small glass plates, or petri

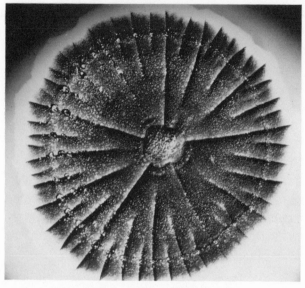

The mold Penicillium chrysogenum, *the source of commercial penicillin. (Pfizer Inc.)*

dishes as they are called in the laboratory. He had a number of cultures of the bacteria called *Staphylococcus*, or staph, growing in petri dishes. Staph is the bacteria responsible for all sorts of afflictions from boils to blood poisoning. One of the cultures had become contaminated. A mold spore drifting in the air had settled into the staph culture and was growing there. It was the sort of accidental contamination that happens frequently in research. The bacteria culture was ruined, and the obvious thing to do was throw it away, sterilize the dish, and start again. Fleming did not do the obvious, for he had noticed that the area around the mold growth had become transparent. The bacteria there had been rendered inactive and had actually begun to dissolve. The mold, it seemed, was producing a substance that attacked the staph bacteria.

Fleming took a tiny bit of the mold and grew it in a broth. Though he was no expert on molds, he was able to generally identify this one as belonging to the genus called *Penicillium*, a soil mold. Under a microscope the mold has a rather brushlike appearance, and the name penicillium comes from the Latin word for brush.

After he had grown sufficient mold, Fleming began to test it on various types of bacteria. He was able to observe the penicillum destroying bacteria. That was the easy part. Any strong antiseptic would destroy bacteria but would destroy flesh and blood as well. That's why the use of a strong antiseptic is limited externally and cannot be used at all internally. When Fleming tested his penicillum on blood, he found that it left both red and white cells unharmed.

Fleming continued to conduct a variety of successful experiments with penicillium—its bacteria-killing substances now reduced to a powder that he called "penicillin." Yet for a dozen years practically no one noticed. It wasn't that Fleming was working in secret, trying to hide his discovery from the outside world. Quite the contrary. In 1929 Fleming wrote a full description of his work for the British *Journal of Experimental Pathology*. The article didn't attract much attention. Admittedly, the mold was difficult to grow in quantity, so the amount of penicillin available for research was severely limited. More significantly, the sort of chemotherapeutic approach to treatment that was represented by penicillin was not well thought of during the 1930s. There was a brief investigation of Fleming's discovery in the United States in 1932—the mold was identified specifically as *Penicillium chrysogenum*. But still there was little interest, and Fleming had to continue to work alone in his own small laboratory with inadequate equipment and limited funds. The great discovery had been made. The time was not right for it to be recognized.

It took the carnage of World War II to spark a real interest in Fleming's work. The sulfa drugs had already been introduced with great success, so the medical world was ready to consider new and different forms of chemical therapy, particularly anti-infection drugs.

It was an Australian-born professor of pathology, Dr. Howard Florey, who dug up Fleming's ten-year-old paper in 1939. Florey visited Fleming at Saint Mary's and found that he still had descendants of the original mold growing in flasks in his little laboratory. A bit of the mold was transfered to Florey's lab at Oxford, and work began in earnest. Both civilian and military casualties were piling up in the hospitals, and even with the sulfa drugs there was a high death rate from infection.

The first test of penicillin on a human subject came in February 1940. The patient was a London policeman who had cut his face shaving and then developed a vicious staphylococcal blood poisoning. Sulfa drugs were of no use against this kind of infection, and the patient was dying. Florey and his associates decided to test the new drug on the dying policeman. For five days penicillin was administered. The policeman's temperature began to drop. The horrible swellings on his face started to subside, and he appeared on his way to a normal recovery.

Unfortunately, medical research does not always follow the happy-ending script. The great drawback of penicillin was that the body does not retain it, and that in order for it to be effective it has to be administered repeatedly and in massive doses. In those early days penicillin was extremely difficult to produce, and after five days of treating the policeman the supply ran out. The policeman's infection began to spread once again. Florey and his associates tried to scrape together a new supply, but they had too little too late. The infection had grown worse, and the policeman died.

Further tests were tried on patients suffering from severe infections. Sometimes the patients recovered, sometimes they did not. As with the policeman, the major problem was lack of a large quantity of precious penicillin. That problem was solved by scientists working at the Northern Regional Laboratories in Peoria, Illinois. They developed methods of growing the mold in huge metal vats that had been made for the distilling of alcohol. And then, with the commercial success of penicillin looking very bright indeed, the drug companies, which had expressed no interest in the earlier research, suddenly changed their minds.

At first the new drug was expensive and hard to come by. When commercial production began, the war was still on and penicillin was strictly rationed. In 1943, during the first five months of production, 400,000,000 units of the drug were turned out. By the end of the year, the figure had jumped to 9,194,000,000 units a month—and that was just the beginning. In late 1948, eight million million units of pure crystalline penicillin were rolling out of the laboratories every month.

Penicillin was the first of a long list of antibiotics—bacteria-fighting drugs made from living organisms—that were produced over the next decade or so. Penicillin was also the first product to which the term "wonder drug" was widely applied. And as the public became acquainted with penicillin in the years following World War II, it seemed like a wonder. There had been tales of how the drug had saved the lives of many soldiers during the war, but now people began to see the operation of this new medical

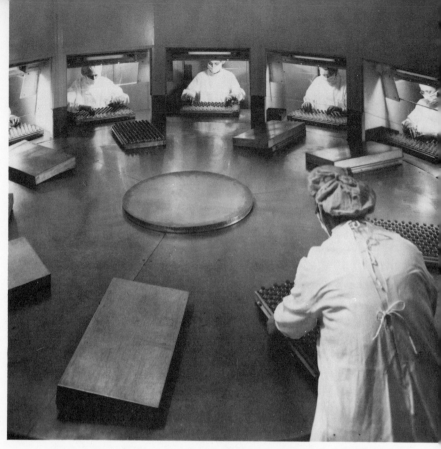

The commercial production of antibiotics around 1949. (Pfizer Inc.)

miracle firsthand. A child with a serious strep throat, who might otherwise have been in bed for weeks and faced the danger of contracting heart-damaging rheumatic fever, could be cured in a matter of days. Oh, there were jokes about penicillin, particularly since injections were fairly painful and usually given in the seat, but people were truly awed by the prospects of antibiotics.

The ever-increasing number of newly developed antibiotics seemed to work against such a wide range of infections that for a time the possibility of a life free from infectious disease appeared within the realm of possibility. With intensive research and perhaps a little luck of the type Fleming had, the ancient enemy infection might be banished forever.

But soon a darker side to the story of the wonder drugs began to surface. Cases of what were first regarded as minor allergic reactions to penicillin, such as rashes and sores, were reported with increasing frequency. And then came the reports of more severe reactions, intense itching, peeling of the skin, sudden swelling, all the way to anaphylactic shock, a catastrophic allergic reaction that affects all of the body's vital functions and is so severe that it can kill in a matter of minutes.

A lot of people were allergic to penicillin, and the more the drug was used, the more people became sensitized to it and the more serious the reaction became. The first injection might result in only a rash, the second could bring on anaphylactic shock. When it first became widely available, penicillin was used almost casually for a large number of diseases, even for the common cold, though the cold is a virus disease and quite unaffected by penicillin. The doctor's philosophy seemed to be that penicillin might protect a cold sufferer from more serious secondary bacterial infections. In any case, doctors assumed it couldn't hurt, but it could. As the number and severity of adverse reactions to penicillin was recognized, use of the drug was restricted.

Even more disturbing than the allergic reaction was the realization that in a very short time bacteria appeared that were resistant to penicillin. Effective though penicillin was, its killing power was not absolute. The organisms that survived were immune to the drug. Some grew more virulent as a result of exposure to the antibiotic. Fleming first noticed the penicillium mold growing on a culture of staphylococci bacteria. By the 1950s there were strains of penicillin-resistant staph, and this sort of resistant staph infection was particularly prevelant in hospitals where penicillin had been freely used. Sometimes these antibiotic-resistant infections were caused by bacteria that had not previously been considered dangerous.

Louis Pasteur, the father of microbiology and the germ theory of disease, had once warned of epidemics that might arise because microorganisms that had been giving no trouble would suddenly be roused and turn vicious; antibiotics occasionally appeared to act as irritants. The dream of freedom from infectious diseases through the new wonder drugs was beginning to turn into a nightmare.

The solution seemed to lie in the development of new and more effective antibiotics that would not produce severe allergic reactions and could deal with the penicillin-resistant bacteria. Some of these new antibiotics, like streptomycin, were in their turn hailed as new wonder drugs. But shortly, the old problems of allergic reactions and resistant bacteria cropped up once again.

The antibiotics were not the only "wonder drugs" in which initial great hopes were followed by unexpected and sometimes crushing disappointments. Cortisone is a hormone that was first isolated in the 1930s. It remained rare and expensive until after World War II, when new methods of production made it widely available. Cortisone was first used to treat rheumatoid arthritis, apparently with enormous success. Arthritics faced a lifetime of incurable and increasing stiffness and pain. With cortisone, people who had been bedridden were able to get up and walk for the first time in years. The effects were miraculous, at first.

The side effects, however, were not easily overlooked. They ranged from women patients who suddenly grew beards, to insanity and heart disease in other patients. Cortisone disturbed the immune system and left many patients highly susceptible to infection. Horrible as the disease of arthritis was, the cortisone cure sometimes turned out to be worse.

And in the end it was discovered that cortisone didn't work as well as had first been reported. Follow-up studies showed that many of the "cured" or "improved" patients had relapsed to their former state of illness. When the British Medical Research Council compared cortisone with aspirin to decide which was the drug of choice for patients with rheumatoid arthritis, the report concluded that cortisone's introduction had "not materially affected the prognosis" and that at least in the first few years "medication with aspirin is more often likely to prove satisfactory than medication with cortisone."

Why had the cortisone tests, and the tests of many other new drugs, appeared successful at first, only to have these optimistic results reversed in follow-up studies? One partial explanation is what is called the placebo effect. A placebo is a pill or an injection of a medically inert material—for example, a coated sugar pill. The patient and sometimes the doctor think that the useless and harmless pill is a powerful new drug. As a result, the patient who takes the pill genuinely expects that it is going to make him feel better, and it does, at least for a while. The mind has a powerful, and as yet ill-understood, effect upon the body.

The placebo effect had been recognized for a long time. But it was only with the introduction and testing of masses of new drugs that its full power was realized. The placebo effect worked not only on the patients, who felt better because they thought they should rather than because the drug had any beneficial effect, it also worked on the doctors, who, thinking they had an important new therapeutic tool at their command, saw improvement where there was little or none. Thus, first reports of uses for a new drug tended to be overoptimistic. More recently a host of complicated and stringent procedures have been devised to screen out the placebo effect from the tests of new drugs.

The greatest medical horror story of the past one hundred years concerns the introduction of a new drug. The drug was called thalidomide, an effective yet mild sedative manufactured by a West German drug firm. In the late 1950s the drug had undergone all the standard tests for safety and effectiveness thought necessary at the time. The tests indicated that the drug was without significant side effects.

And the drug *was* without significant side effects, for most people. But when thalidomide was taken by women in the early stages of pregnancy, their babies could be born grossly, often hideously, deformed. Several thousand such "thalidomide babies" were born in West Germany between 1959 and 1962, and several hundred more were born in Great Britain, where the drug was also in use. The United State was spared the thalidomide tragedy because a government health official just had a feeling that the drug had not been adequately tested and would not clear it for use in the United States, though under existing laws the drug probably could have been marketed.

The thalidomide horror came as a rude shock not only to physicians and drug companies but to the general public. Up until that time it had simply been assumed that an unborn child was protected from the effects of any drug given to its mother, and that a drug safe for the mother was safe for the child. Thalidomide showed that assumption to be patently untrue. The whole medical philosophy regarding the taking of any drugs during pregnancy turned 180

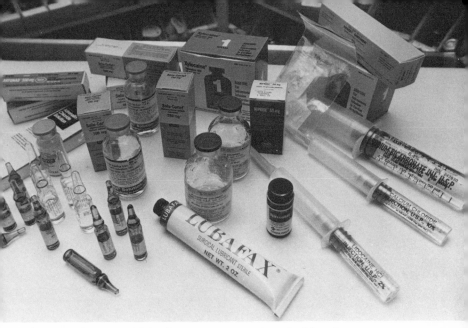

Selection of drugs used in the emergency treatment of heart patients. (American Heart Association)

degrees. After the thalidomide disaster, pregnant women were advised to take no drugs, no matter how safe they were thought to be, except under the press of extreme necessity, particularly during the early stages of pregnancy.

What made the thalidomide tragedy doubly terrible was that the drug was not being taken to save a life or cure a serious ailment; it was merely to relieve mild anxiety.

At the end of the last century, the average physician didn't have a lot of trouble figuring out what to prescribe for his patient. He didn't have a wide variety of medicines at his command. He could carry a fairly good supply of what he needed around in his familiar black bag.

The chemical revolution in drug therapy changed that forever. The modern doctor has thousands of drugs he can choose from, many on the market just a few months or years. Hundreds of powerful new drugs appear on the

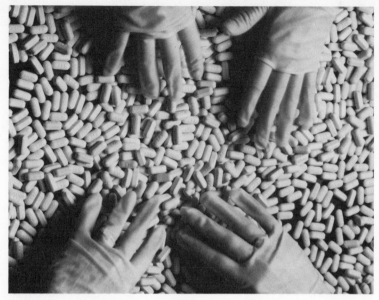

Today the production of massive quantities of drugs is one of the world's leading industries. (Pfizer Inc.)

market every year. The dilemma the physician now faces is that there are almost too many drugs.

Laws and regulations regarding the safety and testing of new drugs have been tightened considerably since the era of indiscriminate use of penicillin and the thalidomide horror. The average physician is more cautious about pushing the latest pill. But virtually all powerful drugs have side effects, effects that may be worse than the condition the drug is being administered to correct. For many, the side effect is really the main effect. Individual reactions to drugs vary greatly. Then there are the problems of combinations of drugs—a patient may be taking five, six, or more drugs at one time. Alone a drug may be useful and benign; in combinations with other drugs it may become ineffective, dangerous, or deadly.

How can the average busy doctor keep up with the vast and ever-changing field of therapeutic drugs? Some critics both in and outside the medical profession say that a doctor can't keep adequately informed and that he or she relies primarily, or at least too heavily, on information and advertising put out by the drug companies themselves. Obviously no drug company wants a thalidomide, but the companies are primarily interested in selling their products. Their information highlights advantages and downplays dangers.

Besides the grave risks of prescribing the wrong drug or a lethal combination of drugs, there is also the problem of prescribing too many drugs, period. Are drugs really necessary for a minor condition or for an illness that will go away on its own? Some doctors complain that they are pushed into prescribing by their patients, who demand a pill for every little ailment or pain. Medical critics insist that sometimes the push is the other way. Doctors give out drugs without adequately informing the patient of the possible ill effects or even of what the drug is supposed to do for them. Some critics have charged that patients are used as unknowing guinea pigs for new drug therapies. The whole area of what drug to prescribe and when, and even if, is one of the most sensitive in medicine today.

There can be no serious argument about the ultimate value of the chemotherapeutic revolution. Many of us would not be alive today were it not for penicillin or some of the other products of that revolution. But like all revolutions, this one has had its excesses. Modern medicine still hasn't fully and efficiently absorbed all of the changes that have been brought about.

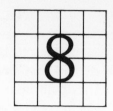

DANGEROUS DRUGS

THE WRITER Robert Louis Stevenson was a victim of tuberculosis. He traveled all over the world in search of a climate in which his frail health might improve. He finally reached the island of Samoa in the South Seas, where he believed he found such a place.

On January 20, 1890, Stevenson wrote a long-delayed letter to his doctor back in Europe:

> My Dear (Doctor) Scott:
>
> Shameful indeed that you should not have heard of me before. I have been some twenty months in the South Seas and I am (up to date) a person whom you would scarcely know. . . .
>
> I am so pleased with this climate that I have decided to settle; have even purchased a piece of land. . . .
>
> Now you would have gone longer without news of your truant patient but that I have a medical dis-

covery to communicate. I find I can (almost immediately) fight off a cold with liquid extract of coca;
two or (if obstinate) three teaspoonfuls in the day for
a variable period of from one to five days sees the cold
generally to the door. I find it at once produces a glow,
stops rigour, and though it makes one very uncomfortable, prevents the advance of the disease. Hearing
of this influenza, it occurred to me that this might prove
remedial; and perhaps a stronger exhibition (might be)
still better.

Stevenson's "cold remedy" is the drug that we now
know as cocaine. In the same letter Stevenson tells his doctor that he thinks injections of cocaine would help ward
off influenza, which was raging in Europe at that time.

Stevenson was lucky. Aside from feeling "very uncomfortable," he seems to have suffered no long lasting ill
effects from his self-experimentation with a drug more
powerful than he knew. Others were not so lucky. The
great surgeon Dr. William Halsted, who was Harvey
Cushing's teacher and one of the famous medical faculty
members at Johns Hopkins, became addicted to cocaine
when he was conducting experiments with the drug as a
local anesthetic. Though Halsted was ultimately cured of
his addiction, many of his colleagues believed that it had
brought about permanent changes in his personality and
made him more difficult than ever to deal with.

It's revealing to look back over the last one hundred
years and see how many drugs once thought to be beneficial, nearly miraculous in some cases, are now regarded
as addictive and dangerous. Many have been declared
illegal.

Cocaine is an excellent example. For centuries many
South American Indians chewed the leaves of the coca

plant, from which cocaine is derived, for their narcotic effect. The powerful narcotic alkaloid the leaves contain is cocaine. The drug itself was first isolated in 1858, one of the early triumphs of pharmaceutical chemistry. By the end of the nineteenth century, the search was on for new, more effective, and safer forms of anesthetics. Researchers naturally turned to cocaine. In 1884 physicians first began using cocaine injections as a local anesthetic, the first ever, and this practice was continued for many years until the addictive dangers of the drug were fully understood. Early in his career, Sigmund Freud, founder of psychoanalysis, tried

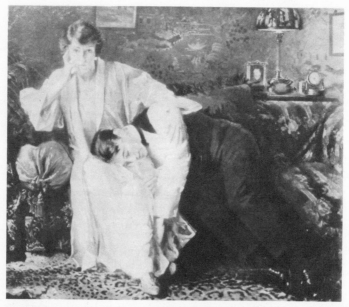

A 1919 *painting by Alfred Priest entitled "Cocaine." (New York Public Library Picture Collection)*

using cocaine to aid some of his mental patients, though he soon gave up the attempt as ineffective.

Even as the anesthetic and other medical properties of cocaine were being explored, it was also being used for other, and older, purposes. Less than a century ago, Western society was tolerant of, or at least relatively indifferent to the recreational use of narcotics, which today provokes a near hysteria. Perhaps no where can the difference between the values of a century ago and those of today be seen more clearly than in the stories about Sherlock Holmes. These stories, which were written at the end of the last century, are still enormously popular today.

No modern reader of the Sherlock Holmes stories can fail to be struck by the fact that the great detective was a cocaine addict.

> Sherlock Holmes took the bottle from the corner of the mantlepiece and his hypodermic syringe from its neat morocco case. With his long, white, nervous fingers he adjusted the delicate needle and rolled back his left shirtcuff. For some little time his eyes rested upon the sinewy forearm and wrist, all dotted and scarred with innumerable puncture marks. Finally, he thrust the sharp point home, pressed down the tiny piston, and sank back into the velvet-lined armchair with a long sigh of satisfaction.

Holmes's companion and chronicler, Dr. James Watson, certainly did not approve of the detective's habit. Watson was continually warning Holmes that it might have bad effects upon his constitution. But then, Watson was always fussing over Holmes, telling him that this or that act or omission would damage his health. In regard to cocaine, Holmes admitted that the physical effects might be bad, but—"I find it, however, so transcendently stimulating and clarifying to the mind that its secondary action is a matter of small moment."

The view of cocaine expressed in these stories represented a medical as well as a popular one. Sherlock Holmes's creator, Arthur Conan Doyle, was himself a trained physician (though not a very successful one, which is why he took up writing). Doyle, like his fictional medical man Dr. Watson, did not approve of the use of cocaine. But he was not hysterical about it, either, and Holmes's late-Victorian readers were not offended by their hero's addiction any more than twentieth-century readers were offended by Sam Spade's heavy drinking. It should be pointed out, however, that in the later Sherlock Holmes stories the references to his cocaine habit are dropped—perhaps indicating a hardening of Conan Doyle's attitude toward using the drug.

A modern writer, Nicholas Meyer, fashioned an extremely clever novel, *The Seven Percent Solution*, in which Sherlock Holmes is shown as a hopeless and hallucinating cocaine addict who seeks the aid of the young Sigmund Freud to help cure his addiction.

Sherlock Holmes was an addict because he enjoyed using the drug. Drug addicts were common in England and America a century ago. Unlike Holmes, most of them had become addicted through prolonged medical use of an addicting drug. It was the doctor, not the pusher, who started the majority of addicts down the road to drug dependency.

Even more important than cocaine in the history of medicine are opium and its many derivatives. In one form or another, opium has been known for centuries, and it has been widely used in medicine. Indeed, at times it has been considered almost a universal remedy, and one seventeenth-century British medical pioneer declared that to practice medicine without opium would be cruel. Heavy medical use of opium in a variety of forms and for many different purposes continued well into the twentieth century. You may recall that King Edward VII's physicians fed the king heavy doses of opium for his inflamed appendix. It was the standard treatment of the time. In the first decade of this century, an authoritative list of the ten most important drugs in medicine ranked opium and its derivatives second, just behind ether and other anesthetics.

The addictive dangers of opium and opium derivatives were known, though perhaps not fully appreciated, by doctors one hundred years ago. But at that time, opium was the only drug around for many, many important medical tasks. Opium and its derivatives not only produced a euphoric feeling but could be used to deaden pain, induce sleep, slow the activity of the involuntary muscles, suppress coughs, and relieve diarrhea and vomiting.

The most medically useful of all the opium derivatives was morphine, first discovered in 1818. By the end of the nineteenth century, aspirin had replaced morphine as the primary painkiller for minor pains. But for more serious pain, morphine remained the drug of choice. It was freely, even carelessly, given out by physicians right through the early decades of this century. As a result, a huge number of medically induced morphine addicts were produced. Using morphine was a great risk, but for severe, prolonged pain there often was no other form of relief. Interestingly, no one really knows why morphine or many other painkillers work. They don't seem to actually block the pain. The user still feels pain, but doesn't care anymore. As with other addictive drugs, the morphine user rapidly builds up a tolerance to it and must have larger and larger doses to achieve the same effect. For short-term control of pain, morphine didn't present any great problems, but for those who suffered from long-term or chronic pain, the use of morphine was highly dangerous.

Ironically, heroin, the most notorius of all the illegal addictive drugs today, was originally developed by the giant Bayer company as a cure for morphine addiction. It was called "heroin" because of its supposedly "heroic" qualities in fighting addiction!

Dr. Watson may have disapproved of his friend Sherlock Holmes's use of cocaine, but he freely prescribed laudanum to his patients who had trouble sleeping. Laudanum, which had been known for hundreds of years, enjoyed a great surge of popularity as a "sleeping powder" during the late nineteenth and early twentieth century. Its active ingredient is opium, and like other opium products, laudanum is addictive over a period of time.

Another opium derivative is codeine, which can be used as a mild painkiller but was most commonly employed in syrups as a cough suppressant. Long after other opium-based medicines were either eliminated or rigorously controlled, codeine cough syrups were easily available even for children, for they were not thought to be addictive. However, restrictions on the use of codeine in medicine have become increasingly strict since the early 1960s.

In our drug-conscious environment, it is difficult to realize that less than a century ago addictive narcotics like opium and cocaine were the primary active ingredients in many popular patent medicines. The medicines worked

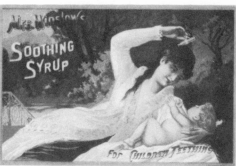

Some examples of nineteenth-century advertising of "cures" for morphine and opium addicts. Some of the causes of addiction are seen in two other ads. Dr. Ayer's Cherry Pectoral (left) contained heroin, and Mrs. Winslow's Soothing Syrup (right) contained a grain of morphine per ounce. It was to be given to teething children. (New York Public Library Picture Collection)

because the drugs killed pain, put people to sleep, or produced a euphoric feeling—but they did not cure anything.

Around the turn of the century, people who bought products like Mrs. Winslow's Soothing Syrup in the corner drugstore probably didn't know that what was really soothing them was a heavy dose of morphine contained in the syrup. Such syrups were commonly marketed for infants to ease "colic" or teething pain. No wonder the infants were "soothed."

Yet there were virtually no regulations controlling the sale of such dangerous patent medicines. Medicine manufacturers insisted that any form of regulation represented an infringement on their freedom to do business. Around the turn of the century, there may have been 200,000 addicts in the United States. Most of the addiction resulted from taking the medicines of the day, either patent medicines or prescription drugs.

But the attack on the medical use of narcotics had begun. In a landmark series of exposés that appeared in the magazine *Colliers* in 1905, Samuel Hopkins Adams attacked the entire patent-medicine field. He was most bitter toward the manufacturers of "catarrh powders" that contained cocaine and soothing syrups that contained opium. It was a "shameful trade," he asserted, "that stupefies helpless babies and makes criminals of our young men and harlots of our young women."

The patent-medicine manufacturers had successfully blocked any form of regulation for a quarter of a century, but by 1905 the mood of the country was different, and, fearing federal regulation, the manufacturers began to cut down the percentage of narcotics and alcohol in some of their products voluntarily. But they didn't eliminate these ingredients, and they continued to resist government regulation. Regulation finally came in 1914 in the form of the Harrison Narcotic Act, which placed a ceiling on the amount of narcotics and alcohol in patent medicines. In addition to getting people hooked on addictive drugs, patent-medicine manufacturers also sold worthless addiction "cures."

Though the percentage of narcotics in patent medicines was limited after 1914, narcotics were certainly not eliminated. It wasn't until 1938 that manufacturers even had to warn users of such potions that the medicines contained ingredients that "might be habit-forming."

In the years following World War I, the dangers of narcotics were recognized throughout the world, and first under the League of Nations and later under the United Nations there were efforts to control the international trade in drugs like cocaine and opium. In most countries the legitimate medicinal uses of these drugs were cut back sharply as they were replaced by other less habit-forming products. Even semilegitimate uses in patent medicines were reduced and ultimately eliminated.

In the early years following the passage of the Harrison Narcotics Act, drug addiction was still treated as a medical problem. The addicts were in the hands of individual doctors or public clinics. However, attitudes in the country were changing. Addiction came to be looked on more as a criminal than a medical problem. Most doctors didn't really try to treat an addict, they just maintained him or her by providing an adequate supply of narcotics. As a result, many doctors were arrested, and several thousand were jailed or lost their medical licenses for dispensing narcotics. Doctors became unwilling to prescribe narcotics to addicts, and the public clinics that also dispensed narcotics were closed. Since drug addiction itself came to be considered a criminal offense, the addict was now sent to jail rather than to a hospital.

The hard-line nonmedical approach to drug addiction seemed to work; the number of addicts fell rapidly. But there was a certain percentage of the addicted population who either couldn't or wouldn't kick their habits. These addicts automatically became criminals because they had to obtain their drugs through illegal sources, and they often had to steal to get the money for the increasingly expensive drugs. While the total number of drug addicts in the

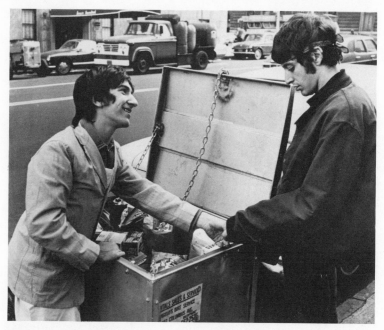

Scene from The Panic in Needle Park, *a grim film about drug addiction. The young addict is played by Al Pacino (right). (Twentieth Century-Fox)*

United States fell between the start of World War I and the end of World War II, after that it began to rise again. There are not as many people addicted to opium products in the United States today as there were back in 1900, yet drug addiction probably represents a more serious medical and social problem than it ever has. Today's heroin addict is different from the typical medically created morphine addict of a century ago, and his addiction is much harder to treat.

Another drug problem that arose during the past one hundred years concerns the psychoactive or hallucinogenic drugs. There are a whole variety of such drugs that occur in nature. Many of them had been used by peoples throughout the world, particularly by the Indians of South and Central America, for their consciousness-altering properties. But psychoactive drugs had never been widely used in the United States or Europe, except in certain artistic circles. Nor were such drugs thought to have any beneficial medical effects. The whole view of phychoactive drugs changed with the introduction of a powerful new synthetic drug, lysergic acid diethylamide, or LSD, during the 1950s.

LSD was first synthesized in 1934, but its psychological effects were not noticed until 1938, when a Swiss researcher, Albert Hofmann, took a small quantity of the drug and experienced, "a not unpleasant state of drunkenness which was characterized by an extremely stimulating phantasy." Research with the drug was suspended during the war years, but after the war it began once again, and some researchers came to believe that LSD could be used to treat, or at least to study, certain forms of mental illness. Initial reports also indicated that the drug might be helpful in treating alcoholism and drug addiction, reversing criminal behavior, aiding the mentally retarded, and easing the mental anguish of terminal cancer patients. Stories began to emerge of persons who had taken LSD and through their drug experience had been able to confront and solve difficult personal problems. It began to sound as though LSD could serve as a sort of wonder drug of the mind.

Non-medical elements of society also adopted the drug. Soon LSD and other psychoactive chemicals became part of a "movement," very nearly a religion. People reported glowing tales of transcendental experiences obtained through the use of LSD. But there were other stories, stories of horrible nightmarish LSD trips and the bizarre and dangerous behavior of individuals under the influence of the drug. There were hints that the drug might cause permanent mental or genetic damage.

During the 1960s LSD was no longer a medical or scientific issue; it became a political and cultural one. The fierce emotions the controversy generated led to a nearly complete ban on the use of the drug, not only as a tool for individual "conscious altering" but for legitimate research as well. LSD may have genuine medical value, but passions will have to cool before a calm and rational approach to this and other psychoactive drugs can prevail. That is not likely to happen soon.

At about the time American society had become deeply concerned about the problems caused by drugs like opium and cocaine, a new drug problem was growing almost unnoticed. As with opium and cocaine, the problem began with legal drugs, and the dimensions of the problem were not recognized until thousands were either addicted or seriously dependent on the drugs and had to obtain them illegally.

This new drug problem was really an outgrowth,

perhaps an inevitable one, of the chemical revolution in medicine. After the limitations and dangers of opium and cocaine were recognized, the medical profession and the drug industry began to look around for other, less dangerous drugs that might serve some of the same purposes. The drugs chosen to fill these needs were the barbiturates. Medically, barbiturates have been used to calm people and in larger doses to put them to sleep. The first barbiturate was derived from barbituric acid in 1903 and marketed under the name Veronal. Since then there have been thousands of derivatives synthesized, and about a dozen have been widely sold as sedatives or sleeping pills.

For a long time it was not even recognized that barbiturates were addictive drugs. The addiction develops much more slowly than it does with the opiates. It is possible for an individual to take barbiturate sleeping pills or tranquilizers at a moderate level for a long period of time without becoming addicted or realizing that he or she is addicted. Once addicted, however, an individual is in serious trouble, because withdrawal from barbiturates is even more painful and potentially lethal than that from heroin. Barbiturates are also extremely dangerous when taken in conjunction with alcohol, and this combination has resulted in a large number of accidental deaths. No one is really sure how many accidental barbiturate overdose deaths occur every year in the United States; estimates run into the thousands. An overdose of barbiturate sleeping pills has been a common method for committing suicide; about 75 percent of all drug-related suicides involve barbiturates.

The other class of drugs that have come to create great problems is the amphetamines. While the barbiturates slow you down and put you to sleep, the amphetamines speed you up and keep you awake. Medically, amphetamines are used to alleviate depression and fatigue and as an aid to weight loss. During World War II large doses of amphetamines were given to GIs to keep them going without sleep. Amphetamines are not physically addictive, and apparently small doses of amphetamines can be taken over a long period of time by most individuals without any harm. But a huge illegal market in amphetamines has developed. The drugs are taken—illegally—by long-distance truck drivers who want to stay awake (though the drug may cut down on their driving judgment), students trying to cram for examinations, tired businessmen, and depressed homemakers. Even at low dosages, unsupervised use of amphetamines can be dangerous.

During the late 1960s amphetamines became a popular "street drug," because by injecting huge quantities of the substance a user could get a "rush," that sudden feeling of euphoria users of other drugs seek. At this level amphetamines, or "speed," are disastrous, physically and mentally. The dangers of speed became so well known that many "speed freaks" switched to heroin; that drug created fewer problems and the letdown from a "high" was not as severe.

While the dangers of barbiturates and amphetamines became known only slowly, many people have charged that the medical profession in general responded to these dangers even more slowly, and that doctors continue to prescribe the drugs too freely.

One of the most frequent charges leveled against modern doctors is that they overprescribe drugs for minor or self-limiting ailments like insomnia and mild depression. This, charge the critics, has led to a widespread acceptance of the idea that there is a pill for every ailment or negative feeling. We have, say the medical critics, become a "pill popping" society. In the view of the critics, a large part of the blame lies with the drug companies, which push their highly profitable but dangerous and not always useful products on doctors through extensive advertising and highly persuasive sales representatives.

Today controls on barbiturates and amphetamines are far stricter than they were in the 1950s and 1960s, when a single sleeping pill prescription could be refilled indefinitely. However, a thriving black market in both of these classes of drugs continues to exist.

Today most doctors are far more cautious in prescribing barbiturates and amphetamines than they were in the recent past. But the dilemma of when, and even if, such drugs should be used is still with us.

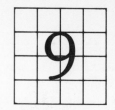

THE MEDICINE SHOW

THE MEDICINE SHOW is part of American history. Picture a dusty little frontier town. A brightly painted wagon rumbles in and stops in the center of town. A small stage is set up in front of the wagon and a man in a frock coat and top hat, who calls himself "professor," steps up on the stage. In a loud and well-polished voice he encourages the townsfolk to gather round. When they do they are treated to a bit of entertainment, perhaps a juggler or dancer who travels with the show. When the audience is big enough, the professor delivers the pitch. He has a "secret elixir," just one bottle of which will cure whatever ails you and restore your youthful vigor. There is a lot of mumbo jumbo about ingredients, some impressive-sounding testimonials, and the elixir begins to sell briskly to the folks at a dollar a bottle. When he is finished, the professor rolls his show on to the next town, while the people in the

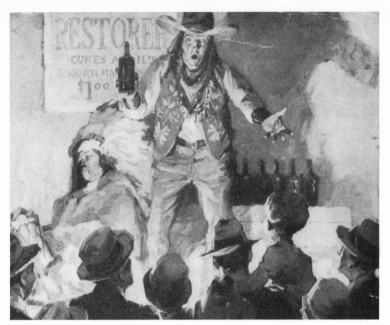

"Step Up, Ladies and Gents" is artist *William Meade Prince's* conception of the old-time medicine show. (Parke, Davis & Company)

previous town are left with bottles of evil-tasting liquid that is good for nothing at all.

The scene sounds so old-fashioned that one could almost become nostalgic about it. Surely this sort of medicine show could not have played an important role in the last century? Yet updated versions of the old American tradition have flourished during the last century despite the great advances in medicine, the stern warnings of medical professionals, and the regulations of federal, state, and local governments. In fact, what was the gaudiest example ever of the old-time medicine show blossomed during the early 1950s.

The product was called Hadacol; the inventor and chief promoter was a state senator from Louisiana, Dudley J. LeBlanc. LeBlanc said that he had first obtained the formula for Hadacol from an unnamed doctor but later improved on it himself. The product was mixed in big barrels behind LeBlanc's Abbeville, Louisiana, barn, and sold for $3.50 a bottle, a substantial sum at the time.

LeBlanc had dabbled both in politics and patent medicine for years before coming up with his big success. Trouble with the Food and Drug Administration forced him to abandon his popular Happy Day Headache Powders, and it was then that he turned to Hadacol. The name was a contraction of the Happy Day Company, plus *L* for LeBlanc.

What was Hadacol supposed to do for you? At first, while it was still primarily a product that sold in the rural South, the claims were expansive. LeBlanc published testimonials to how his wonder elixir had cured anemia, arthritis, asthma, diabetes, epilepsy, heart trouble, high and low blood pressure, gallstones, paralytic stroke, tuberculosis, and ulcers, just to name a few of the serious ailments Hadacol was said to help. Later, as the market for the product reached beyond the rural South, it came under the watchful eye of several different government agencies in charge of regulating the sale and advertising of medicines. Then Hadacol claims were toned down considerably. To avoid laws against false advertising, Hadacol advertising became very vague. Said one critic, "As far as promises went, Hadacol was now good for what ailed you, if what ailed you was what Hadacol was good for."

Hadacol advertising implied, though it never exactly said, that no matter what you had that was making you feel bad, Hadacol would make you feel better. Sales really relied heavily on word of mouth, the whispered rumor that someone knew of someone else's cousin who had been cured of cancer or had his sexual potency restored by generous ingestion of Hadacol. And in case you think that the only victims of this outrageous scam were poor and uneducated southern farmers, you're wrong. By 1950 Hadacol was grossing at least $20 million throughout twenty-two states. It was selling briskly in New York, Chicago, and Los Angeles, and taking in more money than any other medicine of its type in the world. The sophisticated as well as the unsophisticated fell for it.

A good percentage of Hadacol sales could be accounted for by LeBlanc's energetic and clever promotion and saturation advertising. He was spending $1 million a month on advertising. But apparently there were a lot of people who were convinced that Hadacol made them feel better and was good for them.

Hadacol contained a number of vitamins and minerals, dilute hydrochloric acid, honey, and about 12 percent alcohol. There were accusations that the real secret to Hadacol lay in its alcohol, and that people who would not normally drink any alcoholic beverages were getting their kicks from Hadacol. LeBlanc would laughingly brush aside such accusations, though highly alcoholic "boozers" and "bracers" occupied a prominent place in the history of American patent medicines. Many of the "medicine tonics" so beloved by nineteenth-century Americans were really just alcoholic beverages marketed under a respectable-sounding name. LeBlanc, however, insisted that wine had a greater alcoholic content. Wine was also cheaper and certainly tasted better. Hadacol had a rather unpleasant taste and odor.

The accusations persisted, and there were rumors

that teenagers who could not legally buy liquor were getting drunk on Hadacol that they were able to purchase legally in the drugstore. The Chicago suburb of Northbrook passed an ordinance forbidding the sale of Hadacol in any retail outlet other than a licensed liquor store.

Senator Dudley J. LeBlanc himself, was an ebullient and disarming figure. When he appeared on a televised quiz show hosted by Groucho Marx, he was asked what Hadacol was good for. Beaming benevolently, he replied that it "was good for five and a half million for me last year."

LeBlanc really did revive the old-fashioned medicine show, but he had more than a wagon, a stage, and a juggler. In the summer of 1950 LeBlanc's medicine show, consisting of a caravan of 130 vehicles, including steam calliopes, toured 3,900 miles through the South, making one-night stands in eighteen cities. Admission was a Hadacol box top. A dixieland band played "Hadacol Boogie" and "Who Put the Pep in Grandma?" There were plenty of big-name performers on the stage, too. Mickey Rooney, Roy Acuff, Minnie Pearl, along with George Burns and Gracie Allen, were among those who took part in the Hadacol medicine show tour. A West Coast tour the following year featured Judy Garland and Groucho Marx.

For a while the country went a little Hadacol crazy. There was an epidemic of Hadacol humor, and old jokes that related to sexual prowess were revamped with the Hadacol label. Many of those jokes turned up in LeBlanc's road show.

LeBlanc had become so famous that in 1952 he dusted off his old political ambition of becoming governor of Louisiana. He promoted himself as a humanitarian and a statesman and said that his invention of Hadacol was just another of his many contributions to the well-being of humanity.

LeBlanc was challenging the powerful political machine run by the Long family. Though the Longs had controlled Louisiana politics for many years, LeBlanc's challenge must have worried them, because they came up with their own patent medicine, Vita-Long.

This political-medical campaign would doubtless have added an interesting chapter to the history of American politics, if not medicine, but it never quite came off. In the summer of 1952 LeBlanc announced quite unexpectedly that he had sold Hadacol to some northern businessmen. The price was $8 million, and that seemed astonishingly low for Hadacol, which according to LeBlanc had annual sales of nearly $75 million.

The Yankees may have thought they had a good deal and had put one over on the unsophisticated fellow from the swamps of Louisiana, but when the deal was signed and they sat down to examine the books, the Yankees found that they were the ones who had been taken. Hadacol was not nearly as profitable as LeBlanc had suggested it was. In fact, the whole operation had been disastrously overextended, and Hadacol went bankrupt within a few months. LeBlanc had shrewdly escaped the financial collapse by selling out first. He still had his problems with the Federal Trade Commission over his advertising and the Internal Revenue Bureau over his taxes. The sale and revelation of the poor financial condition of Hadacol killed LeBlanc's political hopes. When the election was held, LeBlanc wound up in seventh place.

All of this foolishness, may I remind you, really did

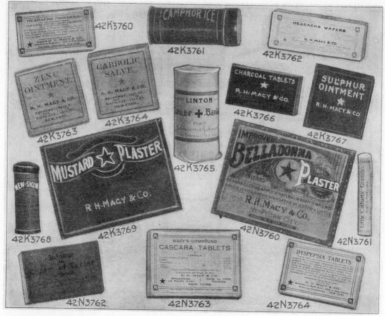

A selection of the patent medicines offered by Macy's in 1909.
(New York Public Library Picture Collection)

take place, and not back in 1850 either. In 1950 hundreds of thousands of Americans were putting down good money and gulping down a musty-tasting liquid in the hope and belief that it would cure them of something. This despite the fact that medical authorities were virtually unanimous in their condemnation of LeBlanc's potion and warned that taking Hadacol instead of seeking proper medical care could be genuinely dangerous. A lot of people didn't believe what the experts told them.

A century ago the first line of defense for most people when faced with an illness was self-medication, often in the form of patent medicines. The term comes from

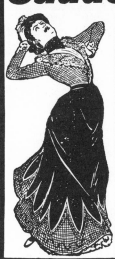

A patent medicine ad. (New York Public Library Picture Collection)

the fact that the formulas for some of these medicines were patented. In reality, however, most patent medicines were not patented, for once a medicine was patented, its ingredients had to be listed. Medicine makers didn't like that. Some claimed that they didn't want their "secret" formulas to become public knowledge. It is far more likely that they did not wish people to know the cheap and worthless ingredients contained in their high-priced concoctions.

The once popular Radam's Microbe Killer, for example, was 99.381 percent water. The tiny remainder consisted of two different acids and red wine for coloring. The solution was utterly useless as a microbe killer, yet it made a rich man out of its inventor, a former Texas gardener named William Radam. In the late nineteenth century it was peddled as a cure for all diseases.

Dr. Rupert Wells pushed a product called Radol, which was supposed to contain the newly discovered radium. In fact it contained virtually no radium and thus was of no value in treating cancer, which was what it was supposed to do. It was probably a good thing that it contained very little radium, for radium can cause cancer more easily than it can cure it.

Microbe Killer and Radol were at least harmless. Many patent medicines, including a large variety of "soothing syrups" for babies, contained cocaine, opium, and other addictive drugs. They were much worse than nothing at all.

In 1905 *Colliers* magazine ran a series of articles on patent medicines. The articles were written by Samuel Hopkins Adams, who spelled out the extent of the problem in his opening paragraph:

> Gullible America will spend this year some seventy-five million dollars in the purchase of patent medicines. In consideration of this sum it will swallow huge quantities of alcohol, an appalling amount of opiates and narcotics, a wide assortment of varied drugs ranging from powerful and dangerous heart depressants to insidious liver stimulants; and far in excess of other ingredients, undiluted fraud. For fraud, exploited by the skillfulest of advertising bunco men, is the basis of the trade.

Attempts to regulate the enormous business in fraudulent and dangerous medicines did not really begin until the passage of the Pure Food and Drug Act in 1906.

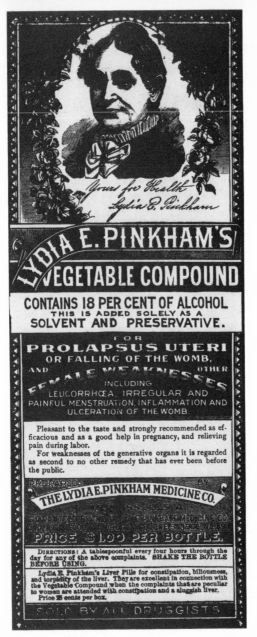

This package, disclosing the alcoholic content, appeared after medicine labels were toned down by federal legislation. (New York Public Library Picture Collection)

Up to that time the medicine men could sell pretty much anything they wanted. Even after 1906 regulatory efforts proceeded very slowly until the late 1930s. The beginning of the century was a time of untrammeled free enterprise. The prevailing ethic was that no one had a right to regulate what business sold or how these products were advertised. The Great Depression, the election of Franklin D. Roosevelt, and the New Deal changed that thinking. New laws about labeling, advertising, and safety were passed. But the patent-medicine business did not wither away. It reformed a bit and adapted. It adapted so well that many of the nostrums used before the turn of the century are still with us today, though often under different guises.

Perhaps the purest survivor is Lydia E. Pinkham Vegetable Compound. Originally it was advertised as a cure for "female troubles." Like Hadacol, the original Lydia Pinkham contained a high percentage of alcohol. The formula has changed, and so has the advertising, but Lydia Pinkham can still be found in many large drugstores, and the package looks pretty much the same as it did a century ago.

Listerine has been more adaptable. It was first marketed in the late nineteenth century as "the best antiseptic for both internal and external use." It was named after Baron Joseph Lister, one of the pioneers in antiseptic surgery. Among other things, the manufacturers recommended it for the treatment of gonorrhea. During the 1920s this approach had to be changed, and Listerine was hailed as a cure for "halitosis," a scary word for bad breath. Listerine also continued to advertise itself as an effective preventive against colds and the flu until the 1970s, when the company agreed to halt this line of advertising in the face of repeated government objections and scientific evidence that it didn't work.

Today the potent and dangerous patent medicines are virtually gone from the over-the-counter market. But there remain a huge number of potions, pills, rubs, and so on, from diet aids to cold tablets, that are of dubious value at best. While the advertising of over-the-counter remedies is much more closely controlled than it was in the free-booting days earlier in this century, medicine advertisers are certainly not obliged to tell the truth. A certain amount of "puffery" is allowed by law, and vague and misleading claims are rarely challenged. Advertisers also exploit marginal differences between products. All aspirins are basically the same—their content and purity are strictly controlled by a host of government regulations. The inexpensive store brand is every bit as good as the more expensive nationally advertised brand. Yet one would not suspect that from the ads we see on television or read in newspapers and magazines.

Most of today's versions of patent medicines are aimed at treating relatively minor conditions, like colds, insomnia, and overweight, or conditions that are not really medical at all, like bad breath and dandruff. The widely advertised bottled cures for serious diseases have been driven from the marketplace. But questionable and downright fraudulent "cures" for diseases like arthritis and cancer have flourished throughout the century and continue to sell well in an underground market today.

Cancer, particularly, has become the chosen field of operation for the out-and-out quack and the misguided medical fanatic. During the past century the fear of cancer has grown enormously. It is by no means a new affliction.

Cancer has been a recognized disease since ancient times, and it appears in virtually all other animals. But as the death toll from infectious diseases dropped, the death toll from cancer did not. It is now the second leading cause of death in the United States. This is primarily because more people are now living long enough to get cancer. But there is also the possibility that there are certain elements of modern life that increase the risk of getting the disease.

While medical science has made great strides in understanding the basic causes of many diseases, cancer still remains a mystery. It is a disease from which no one is immune. The symptoms often appear only after it is too late to really do anything about the disease. Death from many forms of cancer can be lingering and extremely painful. We are almost constantly bombarded by studies seeming to indicate that a host of everyday activities or common household items may contribute to cancer. Medical breakthroughs are announced, and then seem to fade away. As a result of all of this, the public has been left in a state of confusion and fear—a fear that often exceeds the risk of the disease itself.

All is not hopeless by any means. Even if the basic causes of cancer are not understood, there have been significant advances in treating it. Through improvements in surgery, radiation treatment, and chemotherapy, a far larger proportion of cancer patients are surviving for longer periods of time. But the public has not been reassured. Though more genuine and effective treatment for cancer is available today than ever before, there is probably more fear and misunderstanding about the disease as well. The very campaigns aimed at making the public aware of the early signs of cancer have increased the general dread.

People know that despite the endless stream of cancer success stories issued by the various cancer societies and medical groups, there are many cases of cancer which are not curable. Even with the best possible treatment some victims still face certain death. The treatments themselves can be painful and debilitating. Surgery is often radical and mutilating. Cancer treatment can be lengthy and prohibitively expensive. And in the end, after all the pain and expense, it may not work. Cancer patients have often complained that they are treated like guinea pigs rather than human beings.

Small wonder that many patients who have cancer, or people who just fear that they have, are willing to grasp at any treatment, no matter how foolish it may seem and no matter how frequently and fiercely it has been denounced by the medical establishment. The mail order and over-the-counter cancer "cures" have virtually disappeared because of federal laws and regulations of the 1930s. The laws, however, were much less strict regarding cancer "clinics," that is, places where people went to receive unorthodox treatments. Neither the federal mails nor interstate commerce were obviously involved. Control was left up to the states, which typically did little or nothing.

In the 1920s a young man by the name of Harry M. Hoxsey opened a cancer clinic in Taylorville, Illinois, and began dispensing a "secret" anticancer remedy that he said had been developed by his father (or grandfather; the story changed). Ironically, Hoxsey's father died of cancer, a fact that Hoxey went to great pains to hide.

His advertisements ran: "Any person suffering from this malady [cancer] is invited to apply for authoritative information as to the cures that have been effected and are now being effected at Taylorville, under strictly ethical medical supervision, painlessly, without operation, and with permanent results."

In reality there was no medical supervision, and Hoxsey's "secret formula" turned out to be a highly corrosive chemical that ate away the flesh. It could cure skin cancer by destroying the cancer and the tissue surrounding it. Similar corrosive ointments had once been used by many physicians. By the 1920s they had long been discarded for safer and more effective procedures. The Hoxsey treatment could in no way cure internal cancer. Anyone crazy enough to try to swallow the ointment would die.

Soon patients began dying of cancer at the "Hoxide Institute," yet Hoxsey had his supporters as well, and he brought business into the community. At Hoxsey's hometown of Girard, near Taylorville, the local chamber of commerce sponsored a mammoth Hoxsey Day, complete with brass bands and patriotic and religious speeches. A local minister put Hoxsey right up there with George Washington and Abraham Lincoln. But more significant than the bands or the speeches of local worthies were the testimonials given by persons who genuinely believed they had been saved from death by Harry M. Hoxsey's corrosive paste.

The American Medical Association did not join in the celebrating. They called Hoxsey a crude fraud. He threatened to sue for libel but never carried through on the threat. By 1936 Hoxsey had been convicted of practicing medicine without a license and had paid a couple of small fines.

He decided to take his treatments south to Dallas, Texas, presumably a more friendly, or at least less restrictive, atmosphere. By this time he had picked up two tonics, a brownish black liquid and a pink liquid, to go along with his corrosive paste. The liquids were prescribed for internal cancers. The dark liquid contained an expectorant and a laxative. The pink liquid contained substances that helped to control the nausea caused by the dark liquid. While these two liquids did not cause the damage the corrosive paste did, they were of no value at all in treating any form of cancer.

The Dallas clinic was an immediate financial success. It also attracted the attention of Hoxsey's old enemies, the AMA and several federal regulatory agencies. The battle spanned two decades, in the courts and in the press.

Hoxsey's enemies insisted that he was a quack, that the "doctors" who ran his clinic were totally unqualified, and that his treatments were at best completely worthless. They presented horrifying examples of cases in which some of Hoxsey's patients had died when they might have been saved had they sought effective medical treatment instead of relying on Hoxsey's tonics until it was too late.

Hoxsey responded to these charges in a variety of ways. First he presented testimonials from people who said the treatment had saved their lives. Then he said the medical establishment was persecuting him because they feared that their lucrative cancer treatments would become outmoded and that they stood to lose a great deal of money as a result. Hoxsey insisted that he was willing, even anxious, to have his methods of treatment tested by the proper scientific authorities. But he was never willing to agree to a test under the sort of stringent conditions that are used to test most other forms of treatment. He fell back on the argument that the investigators were prejudiced against him and unwilling to look at the evidence that he presented.

There was a political side to his defense as well. Hoxsey allied himself with a spectrum of organizations that distrusted big government, organized medicine, the drug industry, and the food industry, all of which, in the minds of the believers, seemed to be vaguely connected in some kind of Communist conspiracy. It was a conspiracy that was aimed at depriving people of their freedom to take whatever medicines they wished.

It wasn't until 1957 that Hoxsey was finally forced to close down his Texas clinic and get out of the cancer treatment business. Several satellite operations had already closed down. While some health magazines carry occasional advertisements for the raw ingredients from which an individual can make his own Hoxsey medications, this once popular treatment is essentially dead. It had cost the federal government more than a quarter of a million dollars in court costs alone, and it had taken more than thirty years.

The Hoxsey treatment was the best-publicized of the early-twentieth-century "cancer cures," but it certainly wasn't the only one. A cancer drug called Krebiozen, which was brought to this country from Argentina by two Yugoslav brothers named Durovic, rose to prominence during the 1950s. Krebiozen attracted the support of one of the nation's leading scientists, Dr. Andrew Ivy, who virtually ruined his career defending the controversial drug. Though the Krebiozen supporters were in general more respectable than those who supported the Hoxsey treatment, many of the old battles were fought once again. There was the same charge of persecution by the medical establishment and the same constant call for tests but unwillingness to agree on test conditions. And there were the testimonials—above all, the testimonials from persons who believed their lives had been saved by Krebiozen.

Currently the controversy centers around an alleged cancer drug called Laetrile, which is made from apricot pits. Looking over the arguments for and against Laetrile, one gets an acute sense of *déjà vu*. We have been here before.

The manufacture and sale of Laetrile is currently illegal in the United States, but people get the drug anyway. Some go for treatment to Laetrile clinics and other unorthodox cancer clinics that operate just over the Mexican border, where there are no laws to restrain such operations.

The popular actor Steve McQueen, who was diagnosed as having terminal cancer, sought such a Mexican cure. It did him no good, and he died perhaps even more rapidly than if he had stuck to orthodox treatments or had taken no treatments at all. But even such a well-publicized failure will not discourage the desperate from flocking across the border to seek a cancer "cure."

The Laetrile defenders, like the defenders of the Hoxsey cancer cure and countless other unorthodox or downright fraudulent treatments of past years, have organized into a political and moral as well as a medical crusade.

Over the last hundred years the situation regarding the unorthodox, ineffective, and simply fake medical treatments has changed much less than one would suspect. The sure cures for tuberculosis that were once common are now gone because the disease is less common today and effective orthodox treatments are available. But so long as there are diseases like cancer for which treatment is expensive, painful, and often not very effective, people will grasp at straws. Who can blame them?

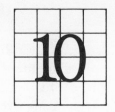

THE DOCTOR'S DILEMMA

THE OLD FAMILY doctor, the general practitioner or GP, the country doctor; the man with the black bag, stethoscope, and kindly bedside manner is practically a mythic figure today. He stands somewhere between the pioneer and the minuteman in the pantheon of American heroes. This figure was nicely evoked by psychiatrist Carl Binger in his book *The Doctor's Job*.

> Time was, and not so long ago, when the family doctor delivered babies and supervised their nursing, their weaning and their teething, when he vaccinated them and saw them through their measles and chicken pox and whooping cough. He told the boy about the facts of life and treated the girl for her menstrual cramps. He advised about diet and rest and gave spring tonic, clipped tonsils, set a broken arm, reassured father who couldn't sleep because of business worries,

pulled mother through a case of typhoid or double pneumonia, reprimanded the cook who was found on her day out to have a dozen empty whiskey bottles in her clothes closet, gave advice about the young man's choice of college and profession, comforted grandma, who was losing her memory and becoming more irritable and closed grandpa's eyes in his final sleep. He went on his endless, mysterious and incessant rounds leaving in his wake a faint odor of carbolic with which he disinfected his beard. This heroic figure is gone from our midst. He survives only in a few remaining rural communities where, like the anachronistic hitching post, he stands as a memorial to our simpler and more rugged past. Nor can our nostalgic longing wish him back into existence. Who killed Cock Robin? What combination of circumstances banished him?

The image of the family doctor is very much like that portrayed in a famous painting by Sir Luke Fides. The painting shows the inside of a humble country cottage. In the background are a weeping mother and distraught father, in the foreground a sick child asleep on a bed made up of two chairs pushed together. And beside her is the bearded and frock-coated doctor. He is the very model of concern, competence, and kindness. You just know that he has been sitting at the child's bedside for hours and will stay as long as required. This picture has often appeared on calendars distributed by pharmacies and drug companies, and has frequently been used in the publicity issued by medical societies.

It is an image that is indelibly planted in most of our minds through books, films, radio, television and advertising. But it is a secondhand image, for most of us

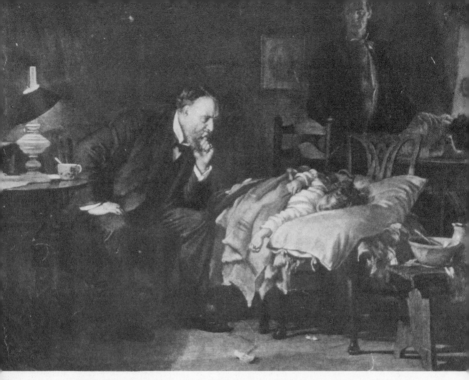

"The Physician" by Sir Luke Fildes. (New York Public Library Picture Collection)

have never seen such a doctor. Still, we are sure that he existed sometime in the past, and we miss him badly. Before we discuss why this well-loved figure disappeared, we must tarnish the image a bit and point out that not every physician of the past was the sort of kindly family doctor we picture. The immigrant living in the crowded and disease-ridden tenements of New York's Lower East Side around the turn of the century had a very different type of medical experience, as this description by A. J. Rongy shows all too clearly:

> The practice of medicine among the immigrants was difficult. There was no family practice. It simply consisted of calls to visit the sick. It was not at all uncommon for a family to have three or four different

doctors a day during a critical illness. Each doctor in turn threw away the medicine prescribed by the previous doctor, made a new diagnosis, and prescribed a "sure cure." If the patient's condition did not improve rapidly, the family became hysterical and insisted upon calling a "professor" from uptown. The East Side, therefore, became a fertile field for consultants. Jew and Gentile alike. The consultation work flourished and every budding specialist made a bid for consultations on the East Side. . . .

Some of the busy practitioners developed a fine clinical acumen and practiced medicine intelligently. There were, however, a number among them who always groped in the dark. Many interesting tales are told of how shrewdly some covered up their ignorance. A story is told of a busy practitioner who was called to see a sick child and made a diagnosis of pneumonia. Said the mother "But, Herr Doktor, the child has no fever." The doctor quickly retorted: "Ah, my dear woman! Don't you know there are two kinds of pneumonia, hot and cold?" Typhoid fever and malaria were popular diagnoses in those days. The physicians had to establish a definite diagnosis quickly, otherwise they were in danger of losing their patients. One of the busy practitioners on Rivington Street, who made anywhere from twenty-five to forty calls a day, when he became tired of climbing stairways, stopped on the first floor, called for the patients on the floors above, asked them to describe their ailments, and rushed off, telling them that they would find their medicine in the corner drugstore.

One of the more poorly trained Lower East Side

doctors is described in this unflattering portrait by Moishe Nadir:

> He has just opened an office and is waiting for customers. He constantly complains that he is sick. When a patient drops in once in a blue moon, he takes him into the [waiting room] where there are numerous shelves filled with (borrowed) surgical instruments which he doesn't begin to know how to use. He lights up the electric machines with the red and green bulbs and the deafening clatter, and says in a professorial solemn voice: "Your stomach has to be . . . (he doesn't say what) but don't be afraid. You'll come in twice a week regularly, and we may not have to use those instruments." He points to the huge glass shelves stacked with nickel-plated paraphernalia.
>
> The doctor's back pockets bulge with bottles of urine, which he is constantly pulling out together with his filthy handkerchief. He is always telling my applicants that their "water" is no good.

Most doctors of a century or so ago were not as bad as the semieducated quack described by Moishe Nadir. But they were not the all-wise healers of popular mythology, either.

The fact is that a century ago the training for most doctors in America was haphazard at best. Europe had a long tradition of university-connected medical schools with high standards. That type of medical education had never become universal in America. At the turn of the century, America had plenty of medical schools, some of them quite good. But the majority were poorly equipped. Even Harvard Medical School had no stethoscopes or microscopes until after the Civil War and did not require a four-year course with written examinations until 1892. Fears were expressed that students could not write well enough to pass the examinations. At the turn of the century, some American medical schools were still teaching the technique of bleeding, a long-outmoded and dangerous treatment. The most ambitious, talented, or richest medical students went to Europe for their training. Some never came back.

At the bottom of the medical heap were the many private, profit-making medical schools that were little more than diploma mills. At these institutions practically anyone could get an MD degree by attending a few months of lectures by a self-appointed doctor-teacher.

In such an atmosphere an absolute incompetent could quite legally set up in practice. Many did. Even the diligent, hard-working country doctor of legend could be embarrassingly short of up-to-date medical knowledge.

People who had observed how medicine was taught at the better European universities and then compared it to the medical education situation in America knew that something was seriously wrong. The man who put all the criticisms of American medical education together into one comprehensive report was Abraham Flexner, a former high school teacher, who in 1908 wrote a highly critical survey of higher education entitled "The American College." His work on colleges was so impressive that two years later the Carnegie Foundation for the Advancement of Teaching financed a major Flexner study of medical education in the United States and Canada. The final Flexner report was thorough and severe. Many doctors were stung by the criticism, but the more responsible members of the profession recognized the essential truth of Flexner's observations. As a result, the report stimulated deep and essential changes in American medical education.

The most obvious reform was that within twenty years most of the diploma mills and inferior colleges were closed. In 1905 there were 160 medical schools attended by 26,147 "students of medicine," from which 5,606 were graduated each year. A medical degree could be obtained by just a few months of not too rigorous study. By the years immediately preceding World War II, the number of approved medical schools had dropped to 77, all of which offered full four-year courses in medicine. The schools were larger and the total number of medical students and graduates was about the same as it had been in 1905. But the population of the United States had grown greatly in the years between 1905 and 1941. This meant that there were fewer, but better-trained, physicians available to the public.

These changes meant an entirely new way in which medical education was financed. In the old days a medical education, or at least a medical degree, was relatively cheap. But the new medical education was of longer duration and required well-equipped schools and laboratories and highly trained, and highly paid, professional teachers. The fees of medical students went up sharply, so sharply that soon the students themselves could not meet the rising cost of their education. The gap had to be made up by gifts and endowments to private medical schools, taxation for state-supporetd institutions, and a great deal of money from the large foundations like the Rockefeller Foundation.

The Flexner reforms abolished the old apprentice system, which had often resulted only in passing on medical ignorance from one generation to the next. Medicine became a full-time postgraduate university education. The report stressed the scientific core of medicine and the necessity for research. Both these ideas were utterly alien to much of nineteenth-century medical education in America.

Yet an essential, if not the essential, part of a doctor's training still remained his clinical experience—his contact with patients while under the watchful eye and instruction of an older and more experienced doctor. The man who influenced the clinical side of medical education more than any other was Canadian-born William Osler. Osler was a man of wide learning, an excellent writer, a philosopher of medicine who inspired almost worshipful devotion from his friends and associates. Osler himself had a simpler description of his chief accomplishment in life. For his epitaph he proposed, "He taught medical students in the wards." And that he did with consummate skill.

Osler was already well known as a physician and teacher when he was called to become part of the faculty of the newly opened Johns Hopkins medical school in Baltimore. Osler had been highly critical of medical education in America and of what he politely called the "unrestricted manufacture of diplomas." Johns Hopkins was to be something new. The Quaker philanthropist after whom the school was named provided money for a first-rate medical school and teaching hospital all in one complex. It was to be a medical school to rival the best of the European schools. The aim was to attract top-quality teachers and students.

Osler quipped to a colleague, "We were lucky to get in as professors, for I am sure that neither you nor I would ever get in as students." The medical school itself opened in 1889, but full courses for undergraduates did not begin until 1895.

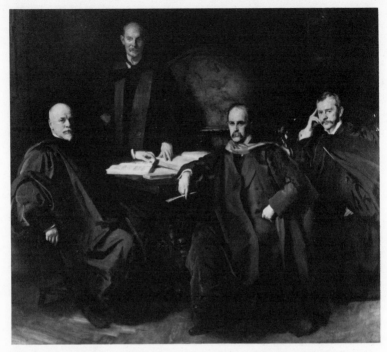

*Some of the original faculty members of Johns Hopkins Medical
School are shown in this famous John Singer Sargent portrait,
"The Four Doctors." They are (left to right) William Henry
Welch, William Halsted, William Osler and Howard Kelly.
(Alan Mason Chesney Medical Archives of the Johns Hopkins
Medical Institutions)*

Osler was appointed professor of medicine and physician in chief of Johns Hopkins, and during his fifteen-
year tenure there his influence spread throughout the country and his fame throughout the world. He ultimately went
to Oxford in England, where he became that nation's
leading clinician and was knighted for his services.

As a writer on medical subjects Osler was without
parallel. His book *Principles and Practice of Medicine*
(1892) was not only an excellent medical textbook that

was the standard one-volume text for decades, it was also a literary triumph. Reading Osler's book during a vacation inspired Rockefeller aid, Frederick C. Gates to suggest to John D. Rockefeller the founding of the Rockefeller Institute for Medical Research. From that day to this, a substantial part of the Rockefeller fortune has been set aside for medical research.

It was on his teaching in the wards that Osler's true fame rested. Osler introduced, or rather reintroduced, the practice of bringing medical students into close contact with patients. Fourth-year students accompanied him on his rounds through the wards of Johns Hopkins Hospital. By all accounts, Osler's thrice-weekly entrance to the wards was a grand affair.

The great man was surrounded by assistants, nurses, and students, or "clinical clerks" as they were called. Osler, always cheerful and encouraging, would sit down at a patient's bedside, listen to what the patient had to say, read the charts, conduct an examination, and then launch into a discussion of the case with the medical students. Those lucky enough to make rounds of the wards with the "chief" always considered them the most important part of their medical education.

William Osler had a definite philosophy about medicine, who should practice it, and life in general. He was always highly quotable. Medicine he said, is "an art, not a trade; a calling, not a business, a calling in which your heart will be equally used as your head." He didn't believe that a doctor's training or life should be narrow: "Medicine is seen at its best in men whose faculties have had the most harmonious culture."

The well-being of the patient was always central to the Osler philosophy of medicine. Medicine, he said, "should begin with the patient, continue with the patient, and end with the patient." And Osler himself was fond of quoting another physician, Dr. Parry of Bath, who said it was "much more important to know what sort of patient has a disease than what sort of a disease a patient has."

Even today Osler is regarded as something of a deity in medical schools. But his advice about producing doctors who have a "harmonious culture" and whose chief interest is in the whole patient has often been lost in the rush of technical training the modern doctor receives.

The old country doctor of sainted memory never trained under William Osler, or in a school that had been reorganized in accordance with the Flexner report reforms. The hard truth is that the legendary country doctor may have been hard working and amiable, but he was also very probably an ill-educated bumbler who ignored (if he was even aware of) the advances that had been made in medicine and treated ailments with regimes long out of date and possibly even dangerous to the patient.

Medicine had changed and so had the nation, but the country doctor had not. Carl Binger, whose description of the old-fashioned GP was quoted at the beginning of this chapter, asked, "What combination of circumstances banished him?" He answered the question in this way:

> To attend to the rather simple medical needs of a family such as I have just described would today require the services not of one man but probably of six: an obstetrician, a pediatrician, a nose and throat doctor, a surgeon, a psychiatrist and an internist. Our question is what forces or circumstances brought these new characters onto the medical stage and led to the

exit of the old-fashioned general practitioner. . . . Certainly the industrial revolution, the great concentration of populations in urban centers, the loosening of home and community ties must all have had their share of influence. But as one looks at the problem more immediately, the outstanding fact is that the new members of the cast we call specialists have acquired each a skill in his own field, a technical knowledge and often a manual skill that no one man can master. . . .

Binger also points out that economic competition helped to force many physicians into specialties. "It became necessary for survival to know something that the other man did not, or at least to know it better."

The general practitioner is not an entirely extinct species in the United States even today. But the modern GP exists primarily in rural and small-town areas, and his or her role tends to be more limited than the old-fashioned GP. The modern GP will treat primarily routine ailments of adults and quickly refer patients to specialists when something out of the ordinary arises. Even in families where the main doctor is the GP, children tend to go to pediatricians, and even simple surgery is handled by surgeons. The GP gives the full range of medical attention only when specialists are not available.

General practitioners often complain that they occupy the lowest rung on the medical ladder and are looked down upon by their "specialist" colleagues. They also tend to earn less money. The GP may, in fact, be a dying breed, but so far nothing has replaced the general practitioner's unique function as the overseer of a family's total health needs.

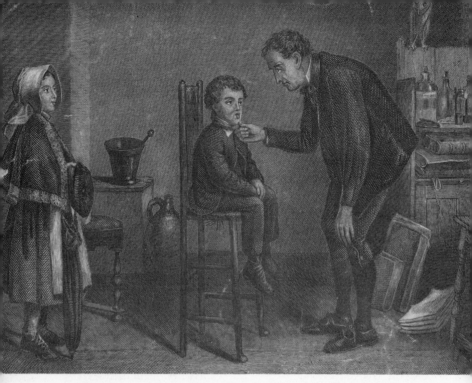

The changing image of the doctor—1870. (New York Public Library Picture Collection)

No one can seriously question the proposition that a team of specialists with all the latest tests and treatments at their command can give a patient service undreamed of by the old-fashioned GP with his black bag. Why is there such a yearning for the good old days? It's not just nostalgia. No one yearns for the good old-fashioned dentist who pulled teeth with a pair of pliers without anesthesia.

At the turn of the century if you needed your family doctor, he came to your home. He might not be able to do too much, but he came, no matter what the hour or weather conditions. The mere fact that the doctor appeared made people feel better. If extended care was needed, he would come back as often as necessary.

Today, typically, the patient must get up out of bed

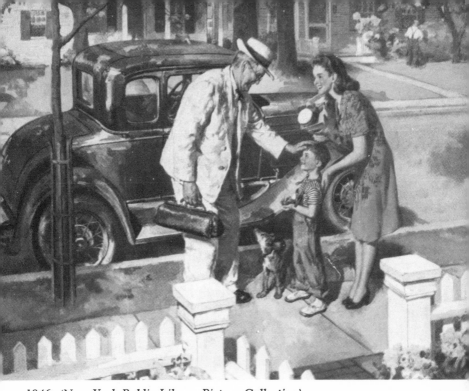

1946. *(New York Public Library Picture Collection)*
Today. *(American Heart Association)*

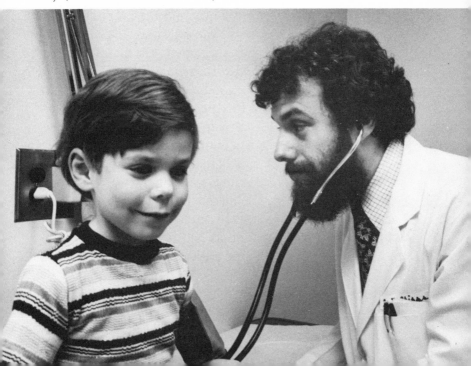

and visit the doctor's office during regular hours. The emergency rooms of hospitals are now filled with patients looking for nonemergency treatment once provided by a family doctor. The patients are forced to go to the hospital either because they have no family doctor or because their doctors are unavailable.

Doctors contend that only in the office or the hospital is there the equipment to do a proper and modern job of diagnosis and treatment. While this is undoubtedly true up to a point, critics of modern medical practice, including many doctors themselves, suggest that schedules are arranged more for the convenience of the doctor than the patient, and that many modern physicians are trying to convert their practice into a regular nine-to-five, five-day-a-week business. The modern doctor is even protected from phone calls from anxious patients by an impersonal, and sometimes downright callous, answering service.

The large cast of specialists also creates a problem. Patients complain that they often are treated as a mass of isolated symptoms by a group that does not really know them as individuals. The complaint has some merit. It is important for a doctor to know a patient and the patient's medical history, even his or her personality, before a proper diagnosis can be arrived at and a treatment prescribed. A group of specialists each working in his or her own area may not be able to get the whole picture, and thus important elements of a patient's illness can be overlooked. There are scores of medical horror stories of patients being shunted from specialist to specialist. Each specialist offered a diagnosis or treatment based on his or her particular area of interest or knowledge, and all of them were wrong because they had too narrow a view.

Money is another serious point of contention. The turn-of-the-century doctor was not a wealthy man. Usually he was no better off than the majority of his patients. Today medicine is consistently the most financially rewarding profession in America. Even in these inflationary times the cost of medical treatment has risen far more rapidly than have costs in most other sectors of the economy. The doctors' argument is that better treatment costs more, and that is perfectly true. It is also true that not all of the rise in price of a doctor's care has been plowed back into better treatment for the patient. Doctors live better, too. Surveys of modern medical students indicate that principal reason a large number have gone into the field is because it pays so well. That is a far cry from Osler's description of medicine as "a calling, not a business."

While late-nineteenth-century medical diploma mills were grinding out large numbers of doctors, there was an oversupply. Doctors had to compete with one another for patients, and this tended to keep prices low. But since the 1950s a relatively small number of new doctors are graduated from American medical schools every year. For a long time there was a real shortage of doctors. People felt lucky when they managed to get an appointment. Without competition doctors' fees tended to rise.

The shortage of doctors in America has been alleviated to some extent by an influx of doctors from other countries. Since doctors in America make more money than doctors anywhere else in the world, a lot of foreign doctors have been attracted here. Are these foreign doctors as well trained and qualified as doctors educated at American medical schools? That is a controversial question. But the fact is that many communities in America, particularly poorer ones, are now served primarily by physicians from places like Singapore, Hong Kong, Korea, India, and South America. Many American citizens who are unable to get into U.S. medical schools go to study abroad and then return to practice in the United States. In 1900, American medical students went abroad to study because they got a better education. Today they go abroad because the schools are easier to get into.

Today's doctors swing a good deal of political clout. The American Medical Association is both a wealthy and powerful organization that can contribute large sums of money to back legislation it favors and defeat legislation it opposes. The AMA insists that its primary aim is to improve the standards of medical care, but critics of the AMA contend that the organization is really devoted primarily to protecting the interests of doctors.

The activities of medical students are carefully watched and regulated by their schools. The graduate of an American medical school is well trained. But once a student gets his MD and sets up in his own private practice, there is almost no regulation or restraint. Medicine is supposed to be a self-disciplining profession. While local medical societies and hospitals do have the right to discipline doctors, this right is rarely exercised. Doctors have a natural reluctance to interfere with their colleagues, no matter how much they may disapprove of a particular colleague's activities. As a result, physicians who are alcoholics, drug addicts, or just plain grossly incompetent are allowed to continue practicing. This may not happen often, but it happens often enough to make the public uneasy.

Patients have retaliated by filing an increasing number of successful malpractice suits. Juries have awarded huge damages, and doctors have begun to complain that they are being victimized by ruthless lawyers and a hostile public. The rates for malpractice insurance have soared. This, in turn, has made the doctors raise their fees to cover the increased cost.

Obviously the modern doctor faces a host of problems that his late-nineteenth-century counterpart did not face. Ironically, some of the most serious problems are the result of the enormous and continuing expansion of medical knowledge. That might not seem like a problem, but how is the average physician to keep up with all the new treatments, new drugs, new rules and regulations? The old-fashioned GP had a small number of tried and true remedies. Either they worked or they didn't. The modern doctor has thousands of new drugs, some of them not very well tried at all. He also has patients who will press him for this or that new treatment or drug that they read about in a magazine or saw used in a TV soap opera. The doctor may feel compelled to overprescribe or overtreat a simple, self-limiting illness because a patient insists that he or she "do something."

In the end, we must conclude that a good bedside manner and a midnight visit are no substitutes for a properly administered dose of penicillin. But the old values cannot be tossed entirely aside. Amid all the modern advances, wonder drugs, and wonderful machines, doctors have to try to retain, or regain, their human contact with their patients, not just as a collection of symptoms but as whole people who have minds and emotions as well as bodies. If that doesn't happen, medicine is not going to be as good as it should, or could, be.

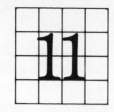

HOSPITALS AND NURSING

On August 21, 1883, a vicious tornado struck the town of Rochester, Minnesota, nearly destroying it. Hundreds of families were homeless, twenty-two people had been killed and several hundred more were injured. Fortunately for the town, the local doctor and his two sons, who were experienced at helping their father perform operations, had escaped uninjured and had lost only their carriage.

The doctor immediately took charge of the rescue efforts. Some of the victims were taken to private homes or to the offices of nearby doctors. The doctor ordered that Rommel's Dance Hall be opened as a temporary hospital. Here the doctor and his sons performed operations, set broken bones, stitched wounds, and even amputated crushed limbs. The doctor's efficiency and skill impressed everyone.

This doctor's name was William Worrall Mayo, his sons were Charles and William Mayo, Jr. The boys were

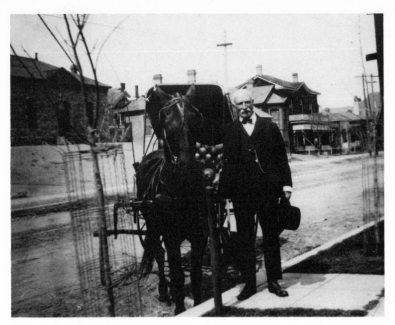

Dr. William Mayo, Sr. with his horse and buggy. (The Mayo Clinic)

soon to receive formal medical training and become surgeons themselves. The Mayo brothers became known as "the surgical twins," though they were not actually twins. Dr. Mayo and his sons did so much for people during the emergency that nuns from the nearby Convent of Saint Francis offered to build them a permanent establishment. Saint Mary's Hospital opened in Rochester on October 1, 1889, and it was the first unit of what was soon to become one of the leading medical establishments in the world— the Mayo Clinic.

But let's go back to 1883 for a moment. What happened to Rochester's hospital? Had it been destroyed in the tornado? No. Rochester didn't have a hospital. Neither did most small American cities and towns.

One hundred years ago the hospital was not as important a part of the medical world as it is today. In America there were a few good hospitals in the larger cities of the East and a number of horrible ones as well. But in general most sick people were cared for at home, and most operations were performed either in the patient's home or in the doctor's office. Only the most severe cases went to the hospital, if a hospital was available, and then they often went there to die.

Traditionally, hospitals were places for the homeless and the poor, who had no place else to go, and were usually run by religious orders. Doctors had little to do with hospitals. People who came to hospitals received no medical treatment to speak of. That changed slowly during the eighteenth century, as the inmates of hospitals received more and better medical treatment. Still, hospitals remained primarily the refuges of the poor, while the better off were treated at home or in private nursing homes or sanatoriums. Doctors used hospitals as training grounds, and the poor patients often served as human guinea pigs.

Many of the great hospitals of today were originally founded as almshouses or poor houses. The horror of such places was vividly described by a late-eighteenth-century French surgeon who complained, "One could no longer see six unhappy patients heaped in a bed, annoying and frightening one another, infecting one another, and one throwing himself about and shrieking when others had need of repose." The dying might be left in bed with the living or on the floor nearby until the next day.

Throughout the early years of the twentieth century, many hospitals, particularly the large city hospitals, remained refuges for the poor and others who had no place else to go. Surgeon Stephen Paget gave his impressions of

a hospital around the turn of the century, and the effect
that it had on a young doctor.

> That is the spiritual method of the hospital; it
> makes use of sickness, to show us things as they are.
> This delicate word sickness includes drink, the con-
> tagious diseases, infant mortality, starvation, the sweat-
> ing system, the immigrant alien, dangerous trades, in-
> sanity, childbirth, heredity, attempted suicide, acci-
> dents, assaults, and all the innumerable adventures,
> tragical or comical, which end in the Casualty Depart-
> ment. To a young man of good disposition, tired of
> the preliminary sciences and of humanity stated in
> terms of anatomy and physiology to the satisfaction of
> the examiners, this plunge into the actual flood of lives
> is a fine experience. Hitherto, he has learned organisms;
> now he begins to learn lives. He need not go, like other
> young men for that lesson, to the slums; for they come
> to him, and that thrilling drama, *How the Poor Live*,
> is played to him daily, by the entire company, hero and
> heroine, villain and victim, comic relief, scenic effects,
> and a great crowd of supers at the back of the stage—
> undesired babies, weedly little boys and girls, hooligans,
> consumptive workpeople, unintelligible foreigners, vol-
> uble ladies, old folk of diverse temperaments, and
> many, too many, more comfortable but not more in-
> teresting people.

Another early-twentieth-century physician, John
Chalmers Da Costa, wrote of Philadelphia General Hospital, called "Old Blockley," one of the first municipal
hospitals in America.

> Blockley is the microcosm of the city. Within
> these grey old walls we find all sorts of physical and

mental diseases, and also a multitude of specimens of those social maladies that degrade manhood, undermine national strength and threaten civilization itself. The sufferers . . . are often the helpless victims of progress. Here is drunkenness; here is pauperism; here is illegitimacy; here is madness; here are the eternal priestesses of prostitution . . . ; here is crime in all its protean aspects; and here is vice in all its monstrous forms.

The language would be a little less flowery today, but the general descriptions given above would still apply to many hospitals, particularly the municipal hospitals of large cities. On weekends, the emergency rooms of these hospitals still are the scene of that drama "How the Poor Live." To the many social and physical ills listed in the statements by Paget and Da Costa, today we can add the cases of drug overdoses, a problem that did not usually reach the emergency wards of hospitals a hundred years ago since addiction was handled primarily by private physicians.

As the complexity of medical treatment, particularly surgery, grew, so did the importance of the hospital. Now even well-to-do patients, who were formerly treated at home, are sent to hospitals, where they can receive better care. Surgery has moved out of the doctor's office into the well-equipped, antiseptic hospital operating room. In hospitals doctors have their patients closer to X-ray machines, testing laboratories, and all the other developments of modern medicine. Any serious illness today is likely to involve at least a short hospital stay.

In the United States three basic types of hospitals have developed. First is the government-run hospital, which can be municipal, county, state, even federal, examples of which are the veterans' hospitals. Typically, these hospitals are large and fill the traditional function of providing medical services for the poor. Then there are the proprietary hospitals, which are run by individuals, often doctors, for private gain. The third type of hospital is the voluntary or nonprofit hospital. These are the hospitals run by religious groups, fraternal orders, unions, or other independent associations. Today, however, most voluntary hospitals, and many proprietary hospitals as well, depend heavily on some form of government support.

The contact of the poor with the large and often impersonal government hospitals was apt to be frightening. In some of the smaller hospitals, particularly those created to serve a particular group, the atmosphere could be quite different.

Irving Howe and Kenneth Libo's book *How We Lived* contains a 1909 newspaper description of Mount Moriah, a small hospital built on the Lower East Side of New York to serve the Jewish immigrants. Mount Moriah is described as a "penny hospital" because it was built through small contributions.

The reporter says, "The entranceway is simple. I felt I was entering a house and was not terrified. An employee greets me with a friendly face. How marvelous this is—I've never been met with a friendly face by a hospital official."

The hospital was a small one, with space for about only seventy patients at a time, and more than half the applicants had to be rejected for lack of room.

> In addition to its own house physicians, patients are treated by visiting doctors from Mount Sinai Hospital as well as by prominent specialists.

> The superintendent was upset that many of the applicants rejected for lack of space felt insulted. Lack

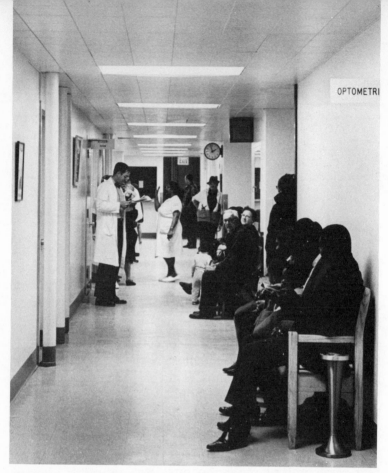

Waiting for treatment in a modern clinic. (Johns Hopkins Medical Center)

of room is not an excuse for a Jew. "What do you mean no room," he retorts. "If you want to badly enough, you'll find a place. I have five children and three boarders in the same four rooms. You push the beds together and squeeze in another."

That the board of health requires a minimum fixed distance between hospital beds means nothing to the father of five and landlord of three. He waved his hand angrily and went off.

Some patients cheat the hospital. A man paid for a private room for a week, then stayed as long as he wanted without paying the rest of his bill. Since Mount Moriah serves no eviction notices, the management could do no more than grumble.

I was given a tour of the various departments. . . . Generally they are as well endowed as the richest hospitals: "all the latest improvements." Except that space is tight here.

Mount Moriah Hospital, about which this glowing report was written back in 1909, has long since vanished. But the tiny hospital out in Rochester, Minnesota, that was established by Dr. Mayo and his two sons has flourished and grown in the most amazing way. The original Saint Mary's Hospital was a small and badly equipped establishment, lit by kerosene lamps. The hospital's water supply had to be pumped by hand, and the sewage system has been described as being beyond description.

Despite all its drawbacks, and its out-of-the-way location, the hospital was an immediate success because of the reputation of its doctors and surgeons. Only 2 percent of the Mayo surgical patients died, an unprecedented safety record. The surgical feats of the Mayos were often reported on the front page of area newspapers. The hospital also established a fee policy that was to prove highly popular. Those who could pay, paid full cost. Those who could not pay full fees paid what they could, and those who could pay nothing were admitted free. But everyone got the same quality of care.

The Mayos were skillful surgeons and equally talented hospital administrators. By the turn of the century they were handling a huge number of operations, 3151 in 1904 alone. Obviously, patients were being attracted from well beyond the Rochester, Minnesota, area. The Mayos had an almost completely free hand in running their hospital and were unhampered by tradition or red tape. Thus they were able to adopt the most modern procedures and come up with many innovations. For example, they enthusiastically and successfully employed all the new antiseptic procedures for surgery. That was one reason why the Mayo hospital had such a low death rate.

Perhaps the most significant contribution made by the Mayos was to develop close cooperation between the operating room and the laboratory. Sophisticated medical testing became the hallmark of the Mayo system.

The money poured in, and the Mayos were able to invest much of it very profitably, and make even more money. The money was eventually plowed back into the hospital, or into what might more properly be called the medical complex, for the Mayos quickly outgrew the small, badly equipped original hospital. The fame of the Mayo brothers soon overwhelmed their ability to handle all the patients who flocked to Rochester. So they established a new type of medical practice. Each patient was seen by a number of specialists and examined with all of the most modern diagnostic techniques and instruments. The final diagnosis was discussed and arrived at by all the doctors. This was the basis for the Mayo Clinic, the first institution to offer private group practice.

Today, nearly eight decades after the Mayo Clinic began, people with ailments that are difficult to diagnose still make the trek to Rochester, Minnesota, in order to be examined by the doctors of the Mayo Clinic. The difference between the Mayo Clinic of today, with its teams of specialists and incredibly complex and sophisticated equipment, and the visiting GP with his black bag, is a graphic illustration of the changes that have taken place in medicine over the last hundred years.

One of the major areas of concern today is the cost of hospitalization. There are about seven thousand hospitals in the United States, and they are big business. Hospital costs have risen faster than practically any other sector of the economy. Very few are rich enough to pay their own way in a modern hospital. Most people in the United States are covered by some sort of hospital insurance, or their hospital costs must be paid by a government program.

The nurse, probably the most familiar figure in a modern hospital, arrived on the scene rather recently. A hundred years ago nurses of any sort were rare. Historically, religious orders took over some of the care of the sick, but they were often more interested in a person's spiritual needs than physical ones. Throughout much of the eighteenth century, most of the women who worked in hospitals were little more than cleaning ladies, and often disreputable ones at that. Hospital jobs were among the hardest, dirtiest, and lowest paying. Charles Dickens's books contain some devastating portraits of these early nurses. The successes of Florence Nightingale during the Crimean War helped to change British public opinion toward nursing. Doctors warned her not to "coddle the brutes"—her patients. The soldiers thought of her as an angel of mercy. America had its own early nursing heroine, Clara Barton, who served during the Civil War. But the prejudice against nursing remained for years in civilian hospitals. One hundred years ago in New York City, women who were arrested on charges of drunkenness were allowed to work off their ten-day sentences as nurses' aids in the wards of

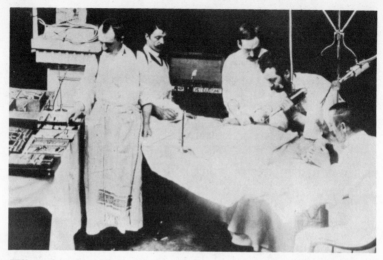

When this picture was taken in 1870, nurses were not yet available to assist in surgery. (New York Public Library Picture Collection)

Bellevue Hospital. They often terrorized and stole from their patients.

But training for nurses had already begun. The medical profession, which had been generally hostile to any form of trained nursing because it felt nursing would interfere with its exclusive domain, had begun to change. Nineteenth-century doctors often argued that women were constitutionally unfit to work in hospitals. A major instrument of change was the gradual acceptance of antiseptic methods. In order to follow time-consuming antiseptic procedures, doctors needed trained assistants, and suddenly the once scorned nurses became a necessity. Once that happened, the doctors decided that women were constitutionally fit to work in hospitals. Nurses began to take over many medical procedures, such as giving injections, taking X rays, even administering anesthesia, that had once been considered the exclusive jobs of the doctors.

The first nursing schools in the United States were established in the 1870s, and by 1925 there were some 2,500 nursing schools. No area of medical practice has expanded more dramatically during the last hundred years than nursing. The first school for women doctors in America was opened in 1850. But the opportunities for women doctors had remained very limited until recent years.

At first, most of the graduates of nursing schools found employment in private homes. The hospitals relied mainly on student nurses, who subsisted on tiny monthly allowances. It was cheaper to use untrained students. But as the complexity of hospital care increased, hospitals were forced to hire the more expensive trained nurses. Nurses also moved strongly into various phases of hospital administration.

In a medical world increasingly dominated by large institutions, we often forget the important role played by the visiting nurse or public health nurse. In the early years of the twentieth century, the first line of health care for many of the poor was the visiting nurse. Visiting nurse societies were set up by the government, by settlement houses, or by a variety of private charitable organizations, most notably the Red Cross.

Visiting nurses were probably more important in reducing the incidence of tuberculosis in the United States than were all the doctors and all the new medical treatments. Around 1900 tuberculosis was found to be a preventable disease. Some tuberculosis patients went off to distant sanatoriums in the country to recover, as best they could, from the disease. The poor could not afford such a luxury, so the tuberculosis patient stayed home, where he was often the source of infection for the other members

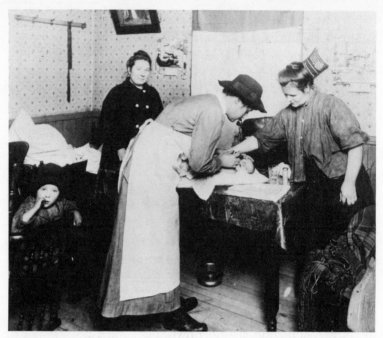

In the early years of the twentieth century visiting nurses were often the first line of health care for the poor. (Visiting Nurse Service of New York)

of his family and the community in general. Visiting nurses were employed to visit the homes of tuberculosis patients and help them institute procedures that would cut the risk of spreading the disease.

Not only did nurses serve the urban poor, they served the rural poor as well. In the areas where doctors were few and far between, nurses often assumed the older role of nurse-midwife and helped deliver babies.

Today nurses are such a familiar and vital part of the total medical picture that it is a little difficult to imagine that a hundred years ago, nursing as a profession barely existed.

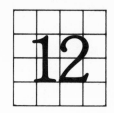

THE FUTURE

Prediction is an uncertain occupation. One hundred years ago someone sitting down to predict the course of medicine over the next century would almost certainly have missed X rays, one of the most significant developments of the last century—and one of the most unexpected. Yet the discovery of X rays came very early in the last one hundred years.

Penicillin languished in obscurity for years before medical science recognized its worth. Then it was widely predicted that antibiotics would end the threat of bacterial infection. That didn't happen either, and few predicted the problems of penicillin reaction.

In 1948 Paul Müller won a Nobel Prize in physiology and medicine for his work on the properties of the powerful insecticide DDT. In the years following World War II, DDT was used extensively and effectively in refugee camps to cut down the incidence of insect-borne diseases.

Later DDT was used to fight crop-destroying insects. It took years before the world fully realized that DDT harmed more than insects. Today this once praised product is banned in the United States and many other countries.

The course of medicine over the last one hundred years has been erratic and unpredictable. The only safe prediction one can make is that it will be equally erratic and unpredictable over the next one hundred. But there are a few areas in which we can expect a major concentration of attention, and we will look at them briefly.

The two biggest killers, cancer and heart disease, will doubtless receive the lion's share of attention from medical researchers. Expensive wars against cancer are launched with depressing regularity, yet the disease persists. Gradual advances have been made in treatment of cancer, but basic understanding of the disease still eludes us. Is there a single biochemical factor that is common to most or all cancers, or is what we call cancer really a collection of different diseases with different causes? The word *plague* was once used to describe a host of different diseases. If there is a single underlying factor, then the control and cure of cancer might come quite suddenly and dramatically, in the same way that the discovery of insulin suddenly changed the world of diabetics. If cancer is more complex, then progress is likely to remain slow and piecemeal. But there will be progress.

There are not likely to be any "magic bullets" to prevent heart disease. No pills or injections that will miraculously clean the fatty deposits from blocked arteries. are on the horizon. Most experts on the heart would agree that the best way to prevent heart disease is through changing certain patterns of eating, exercise, even mental stress. Just what patterns are to be changed, how, and to what

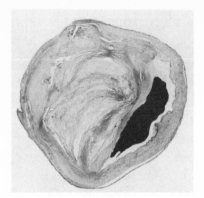

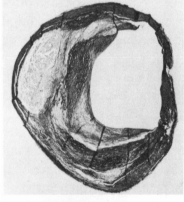

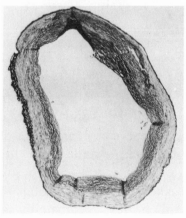

One of the major challenges for medicine during the next hundred years will be the treatment and ultimate prevention of coronary artery disease, the cause of heart attacks. The development of the disease is shown in these photographs. The bottom picture is a cross section of a normal artery. In the center is an artery in which fatty deposits have formed in the inner lining. The top picture shows the narrowed artery blocked by a blood clot. (American Heart Association)

degree are still being discussed, but there already seems to be some success in lowering the death rate from heart disease through this sort of preventive medicine.

In cancer, heart disease, and in fact most diseases, some people seem to be born more susceptible than others. Heredity was once assumed to be entirely beyond the control of medical science—it still is today but may not be forever.

Genetics is now the most active and exciting branch of biological science. Scientists have not only begun to understand just how genes—the very stuff of heredity—work, they have been able, to a limited extent, to manipulate genes in the laboratory, to create and change life.

This area of research, which has been called gene splicing or genetic engineering, has raised the most enormous hopes and horrendous fears. Genetic engineering opens up the possibility of understanding and eventually controlling or eliminating a host of genetic diseases. It also opens the possibility of the creation, by accident or design, of supergerms. The ability to genetically "program" a human being may lie somewhere in the future, but probably not within the next hundred years. Just where we are going with genetic engineering will be as much an ethical, social, and political question as it will be a scientific or medical one.

The ultimate goal, or at least an ultimate goal of medicine, is to delay death. The average life span in America and most of the industrialized world has crept up steadily until it is now a bit over seventy years. Yet it is sobering to realize that the Bible spoke of the span of life as being three score and ten—seventy years. It hasn't changed all that much in thousands of years. The comparison isn't quite fair. For most of history, the majority of those born died in infancy or shortly thereafter. A large number of those who survived were carried off in the prime of their lives by diseases that are now curable. But the survivors reached an upper limit of about seventy. Today a lot more people get to seventy, and a few get well beyond it. But there is no doubt that like other living things the human organism has a definite life span, of approximately seventy years. Science does not now understand why aging takes place or have the faintest notion as to whether the process can be significantly slowed down, but much attention will be focused in that area in the future.

In the meantime, with more old people around there will be greater stress on the special medical problems of the elderly. At the other end of life's scale, medicine has now been able to offer some limited treatment to the unborn. Tests have also been developed that can detect certain serious birth defects early in pregnancy, and no doubt these tests will become more sophisticated and wide ranging as time goes on. If these detectable fetal defects cannot be corrected, what then?

And to return to the subject of dying for a moment, a century ago there was no problem in deciding when a person was dead. Oh, the gravely ill, with no hope of recovery, might linger awhile, but there was little a doctor could do but accept the inevitable and wait. All that's different now. Gravely ill people can be kept alive, without hope of recovery, for months or years through medical intervention. There is no longer even a generally accepted definition of death. This has confronted medicine with more agonizing moral and legal problems that are not likely to be resolved soon.

Mental illness, a subject barely touched upon in this book, will certainly come in for a great deal of medical attention in the future. There is mounting evidence that some serious mental illnesses, like schizophrenia, have a biochemical base, and thus might have a biochemical cure as well. For good or ill, mood-altering drugs have already become an integral part of our society, and their use will probably become even more pervasive as we attempt to cope with that most widespread of all illnesses—depression.

During the last decade or so the problems created by drugs led to a search for more "natural" methods of coping with disease. There was some promising work done in the field of biofeedback—training the mind to control certain "involuntary" body functions such as blood pressure. The enthusiastic initial reports of success with biofeedback may have been exaggerated, but the promises remain. If the complex and powerful mind-body relationship can be more fully understood and controlled, this could represent an enormous advance for medicine.

On a practical level, there are probably going to be some changes in the way medical services are paid for, since medical treatment has come to take an ever-larger percentage of everybody's income. Are all people entitled to the advantages of good medical care, no matter what their ability to pay? This problem is particularly acute for the increasing number of old people, who generally need more (and more expensive) medical care and have less money to pay for it.

One hundred years from now the change in the medical scene may be as great or greater than the change represented by the old-fashioned GP's black bag of a century ago and the dazzling technical facilities of the modern Mayo Clinic.

SELECTED
BIBLIOGRAPHY

Bettmann, Otto. *A Pictorial History of Medicine*. Springfield, Ill.: Charles C. Thomas, Publisher, 1956.

Brecher, Edward M., and the Editors of *Consumer Reports*. *Licit and Illicit Drugs*. Boston: Little, Brown & Co, 1972.

Castiglioni, Arturo. *A History of Medicine*. New York: Alfred A. Knopf, 1947.

Clapesattle, Helen. *The Doctors Mayo*. Minneapolis: University of Minnesota Press, 1941.

Corcoran, A. C., ed. *A Mirror Up to Medicine*. Philadelphia: J. B. Lippincott, 1961.

Eberlie, I. *Modern Medical Discoveries*. New York: Thomas Y. Crowell Co., Publishers, 1968.

Fox, Ruth. *Milestones of Medicine*. New York: Random House, 1950.

Goode, Erich. *Drugs in American Society*. New York: Alfred A. Knopf, 1972.

Gross, Martin L. *The Doctors*. New York: Random House, 1966.

Hibbert, Christopher. *The Royal Victorians*. Philadelphia: J. B. Lippincott, 1976.

187

Howe, Irving, and Libo, Kenneth. *How We Lived*. New York: Richard Marek, Publishers, 1979.

Inglis, Brian. A *History of Medicine*. New York: World, 1965.

Marti-Ibanez, Felix and Sigerist, Henry E. *The History of Medicine*. New York: M.D. Publications, 1960.

Riedman, Sarah. *Masters of the Scalpel*. Chicago: Rand McNally & Co., 1962.

Rousche, Berton, ed. *Curiosities of Medicine*. Boston: Little, Brown & Co., 1963.

Sigerist, Henry E. *Civilization and Disease*. Chicago: University of Chicago Press, 1943.

Spingarn, Natalie Davis. *To Save Your Life*. Boston: Little, Brown & Co., 1963.

Sullivan, Mark. *Our Times*, Vol. I, *The Turn of the Century*. New York: Charles Scribner's Sons, 1926.

Thorwald, Jurgen. *The Century of the Surgeon*. New York: Pantheon Books, 1957.

Wechsberg, Joseph. *The Lost World of the Great Spas*. New York: Harper & Row, Publishers, 1979.

Wise, William. *Killer Smog*. Chicago: Rand McNally & Co., 1968.

Young, James H. *The Medical Messiahs*. Princeton, N.J.: Princeton University Press, 1967.

INDEX